D1083339

Providing
Hospital Services

Providing Hospital Services: The Changing Financial Environment

Gerard F. Anderson
Judith R. Lave
Catherine M. Russe
Patricia Neuman

The Johns Hopkins University Press
Baltimore and London

The Johns Hopkins University Press, 701 West 40th Street,
Baltimore, Maryland 21211
The Johns Hopkins Press Ltd., London

The paper used in this publication meets the minimum requirements of
American National Standard for Information Sciences—Permanence of
Paper for Printed Library Materials, ANSI Z39.48-1984.

Library of Congress Cataloging-in-Publication Data

Providing hospital services : the changing financial environment /
    Gerard F. Anderson . . . [et al.].
        p.   cm.   —(Johns Hopkins studies in health care finance and
administration ; 2)
        Bibliography: p.
        Includes index.
        ISBN 0-8018-3815-0 (alk. paper)
        1. Hospitals—United States—Finance.   2. Hospitals—Protective
payment.   I. Anderson, Gerard F., 1951– .
RA971.3.P78   1989
362.1′0973—dc 19   89-1855
                                                                                    CIP

Contents

Figures
and Tables

Figures

Tables

Foreword

The United States is the only Western democracy without universal health insurance coverage for its citizens. Yet, paradoxically, the United States spends a larger proportion of its gross national product on medical care than does any other industrialized nation. In short, we have want in the midst of plenty—large and increasing expenditures for highly sophisticated technological services at the expense of routine care for the many. These expenditures on technology almost certainly exceed the costs incurred by other countries that provide the services we provide. While American medicine is widely considered the best in the world, and the most technologically advanced, some thirty-seven million Americans do not have health insurance at some time during the year. It is, moreover, uniquely American that health insurance coverage for the poor is organized not as a uniform, national system but rather state by state, with widely variable benefits. Indeed, this pluralistic approach to health care has generated a constellation of payment schemes and service delivery setups, which has had a powerful impact on health providers and consumers in recent years.

In the 1980s, the United States has opted for a free market system in health services delivery, based on the belief that market forces operate the same way in health care and medical services delivery as they do in other parts of the economy and will bring efficiency and restrain prices. This has led to dramatic changes in the health care delivery system. The intensification of price competition, along with payment reform and cost containment initiatives, has the potential to limit the ability of hospitals to provide certain essential services, namely, care for the uninsured, care for high cost patients, biomedical research, and clinical education.

In this book, the authors look systematically at each of these hospital services within the context of new economic forces that are shaping the health marketplace. They focus on academic medical centers, which are responsible for providing most clinical education, biomedical research, and technology development and which bear a large burden of the care of the uninsured. Traditionally, they note, these hospitals have relied on patient care revenues to subsidize unfunded or underfunded services. However, as the hospital sector becomes more price and cost conscious, many hospitals may be unable to maintain their level of commitment to these services.

This book offers readers a new conceptual framework for thinking about the role of hospitals in providing these four services. Taking a fairly unconventional approach, the authors pull these four services together within the same analytical model because of their common denominator: their traditional funding through cross-subsidies, without explicit support from public or private payors. For each service, the authors begin with a brief and interesting overview to enable readers to put current cost and financing issues in a historical context. They offer thought-provoking suggestions for reforming the way in which these services are funded. In the absence of new payment schemes and in the presence of increasingly cost conscious payors and providers, they suggest that there may be no way to support these services in the future: no free lunch. The proposals put forth in this book are in some cases controversial. At a time when hospitals are struggling to maintain their commitment to high-quality patient care, care for the poor, medical progress, and education, proposals such as these warrant our serious attention and have profound importance for hospital administrators, physicians, public and private payors, and patients.

Robert M. Heyssel, M.D.
Professor of Medicine,
Johns Hopkins University School of Medicine
President,
Johns Hopkins Hospital and Health System

Acknowledgments

We would like to thank several people for their help on this book. First, without Robert Heyssel's vision and commitment, this book would probably not exist today. From the book's inception, Dr. Heyssel saw its potential and encouraged us to develop the ideas and pursue the analysis. He reviewed several drafts, offering insightful suggestions for revisions and improvement. We are equally grateful to Steve Lipstein for his continued prodding to make the book clear to as wide an audience as possible. Several other people reviewed the manuscript at various drafts, and we are very grateful for their assistance. In particular, we thank Jim Bentley, Steve Long, Dick Knapp, Craig Lisk, and Karen Davis for their critical reviews, comments, and invaluable suggestions.

A number of people were instrumental in helping us prepare the manuscript. We particularly thank Robert Herbert, the Center for Hospital Finance and Management's epistemologist and programmer, for performing careful analyses from a number of large data sets. Marie Davidson, Loretta Green, and Carole Eng did a superb job of typing, retyping, and correcting the manuscript. We also thank Richard Pan and Christina Johns for their research assistance.

We are especially grateful to those who have worked with us closely to structure and edit the book. Margaret Rutherford was the first to help us pull together the writing styles of the four individual authors. Diane Hammond, our copy editor, helped us to improve the overall presentation and make the document more readable and useful for our audience. We give special thanks to our editor, Wendy Harris, and to others at the Johns Hopkins University Press. Ms. Harris took our manuscript through the review cycle and provided lots of encouragement and support during the rewriting.

Finally, we thank the Commonwealth Fund for funding the project and Margaret Mahoney, Tom Moloney, and Cynthia Woodcock for their support, interest, and enthusiasm.

Providing
Hospital Services

Introduction

The future of health care services in the United States is tied directly to health care financing policies, policies that have changed dramatically in the last ten years. Ten years ago, financing policies were expected to be unobtrusive: they were designed simply to pay the bills submitted by providers. Now, new public and private payment initiatives are beginning to influence what services are provided, where services are provided, how medical practice is delivered, and ultimately who has access to medical care.

These recent initiatives have caused concern, primarily because cost containment efforts have done little to control the overall rate of increase in health care spending. Yet some of these initiatives are beginning to influence the provision of certain services. In addition, there is the potential for health care financing policies to change the health care system dramatically. It is therefore vital for policy analysts to anticipate, monitor, and evaluate the impact of payment reforms on health care services.

Hospitals have been the first health care providers to undergo significant financing reform. Reform of the health care financing system started in the hospital sector for several reasons: (1) nearly 40 cents of the health care dollar is spent on hospitals; (2) expenditures in the hospital sector continue to rise significantly faster than the overall inflation rate; and (3) many health care researchers and policy makers have questioned the marginal value of spending additional resources on hospital services.

In 1980, aside from a few state rate-setting demonstrations, hospitals were being paid on either a cost-based or a charge-based retrospective reimbursement basis. This gave hospitals tremendous flexibility to decide what services they would offer and how much money they would spend to provide these services. By 1984, payment reform had changed the method of financing hospital services, and only a small proportion of hospital revenues were derived from either of these sources. Since that time, the proportion has been reduced further.

1

Since payment reform was introduced first in the hospital sector, it is not surprising that hospital services were the first to be directly affected. One example of the powerful new role that financing policies have on medical practice is the influence of the prospective payment system (PPS) on the care provided to Medicare patients. In 1983, when the PPS legislation was passed, the average hospital stay of Medicare patients was over nine days. One year later, the average stay had dropped by almost two days. The most logical explanation for this change in medical practice is the economic incentive created by PPS to discharge patients as soon as possible. Other changes have been less dramatic but equally significant. The necessity for hospitals to make immediate changes has been dampened by the high profit margins that hospitals have enjoyed during the mid-1980s. This may change if the projections of negative profit margins become true.

Even without a major crisis, the question of how to finance certain services has triggered significant public policy interest, due in part to the immediate concerns of either certain types of hospitals or hospitals in a few locations. To a greater extent, the increasing interest in health care financing is the result of the perceived need to change the ways in which certain services are financed. Those organizations that are paying for hospital services are beginning to become actively interested in what they are paying for and how it is being provided. Hospitals are no longer given a blank check to do whatever they feel is in the public interest. Financing has become a way of implementing public policy.

In this book, we examine how payment reform has affected or could affect selected health care services. In some cases, the discussion of the anticipated effects of payment reform is conjectural, given the relatively short period of time since many of the initiatives have been in place, the lack of an economic impetus to make major changes, and the difficulties involved in isolating the effect of any single initiative on the provision of hospital services. In other cases, the impact of payment reform is more apparent and more easily quantifiable.

We focus on four services that may be more likely than others to be affected by recent changes in health care financing. These services, which have received considerable public policy attention in recent years, are (1) patient care for the patient requiring complex services; (2) clinical education; (3) biomedical research; and (4) uncompensated care. In general, policy debates have focused on each of these services separately. We have adopted a different approach, analyzing the four services within a single framework. Because all four services share common characteristics, a comprehensive solution to all four problems is appropriate. We hope this book will assist policy makers in examining these issues from a common perspective to derive an integrated solution.

The first and perhaps most significant feature common to the four services is that in the past none has been financially self-supporting. Each service has been financed through an elaborate system of cross-subsidization. The production of these unfunded or underfunded services has depended upon the ability of hospitals to generate revenues from other sources, primarily routine patient care, to cover costs. However, as the health care system becomes increasingly competitive and as payors become more able to identify and pay for only the particular services their beneficiaries use, the potential for financing these activities through cross-subsidization is reduced. Because neither clinical education, biomedical research, care for high cost patients, nor uncompensated care are entirely self-financing, they fall naturally within a common conceptual framework. For each, it is therefore increasingly important to identify the costs as well as the external payment source.

A second common characteristic is that these four services are often provided simultaneously. For example, patient care and graduate medical education are produced jointly when an attending physician provides patient care while training residents. During this time, it is theoretically impossible to separate the time and therefore the cost associated with clinical education from the time and cost associated with patient care. Because two, three, or even all four of these services can be provided jointly, any decision regarding the allocation of costs to a particular service is somewhat arbitrary.

A third similar characteristic is that these services are concentrated in a small number of hospitals. Most clinical education, clinical research, and care for patients with complex medical problems are provided in a small subset of the nation's hospitals. Uncompensated care is provided by a somewhat different but overlapping set of hospitals. The future of these services depends upon the viability of these hospitals. Many public and private officials have expressed concern that recent changes in health care financing will jeopardize the ability of these hospitals to provide certain services.

The Impact of Payment Reform on Services

A few preliminary studies have investigated the effect of payment reform on hospital services. To a large extent, concern about the impact of payment reform on hospital services is based more on theory than on empirical evidence (Bergen and Roth, 1984). Definitive empirical evidence is difficult to obtain in such a short time, and the impact is less pronounced, because cost containment efforts have been relatively unsuccessful in controlling health care costs.

From a theoretical perspective, imperfections in the payment methodology could create incentives that would have an adverse impact on patient care. For example, a hospital that is not paid enough to cover costs for certain patient care services may be forced to limit access to certain high-cost procedures in order to survive. Patients with complex medical conditions or patients requiring expensive medical technology are especially vulnerable (Eisenberg, 1984; Omenn and Conrad, 1984). If the hospital is not paid adequately for treating these patients, one of three possibilities may occur.

First, the hospital could provide the care, incurring a substantial loss and, ultimately, going out of business. Second, it could restrict access to complex services or provide lower quality services, and patients having medical conditions that are underpaid by the payment system would be at risk . Third, hospitals may try to circumvent the payment system. For example, in the past, each patient's medical needs would have generally been treated during a single hospitalization; but today, with the changes in reimbursement, hospitals may have an incentive to discharge and readmit patients separately for each condition (Anderson and Steinberg, 1984b; Stern and Epstein, 1985). This in turn may lead to inappropriate readmissions, higher costs, and premature discharges (U.S. General Accounting Office, 1985).

A few studies have indicated that these theoretical concerns may be valid. The American Hospital Association has reported that hospitals are closing in record numbers, particularly those with a disproportionately large share of uninsured and underinsured patients. Several studies identified unintended redistributions of resources by the Medicare prospective payment system (Sheingold, 1988; Feder, Hadley, and Zuckerman, 1987).

Of greater concern, however, are reports that medical practice is changing in ways that are not in the best interest of the patient. Patients are being discharged much earlier under Medicare's prospective payment system than under cost-based reimbursement (Davis et al., 1985) and this may result in discharges that are premature and medically inappropriate (U.S. General Accounting Office, 1985). In a study of patients with hip fractures, patients discharged after the passage of PPS had shorter lengths of stay, fewer physical therapy sessions, and were more likely to be discharged to a skilled nursing home than they were prior to PPS (Fitzgerald et al., 1987). Other studies have examined patients with specific medical requirements, such as those requiring intensive care units (Coulton et al., 1985), parenteral nutrition (Anderson and Steinberg, 1986), or blood products (Munoz et al., 1985), as well as patients with conditions such as cystic fibrosis (Horn et al., 1986) have found a relatively increased risk incurred by these patients under PPS and other payment reform initiatives. Another area of concern involves the diffusion of new technologies (Anderson and Steinberg, 1984a) and medical devices (Foote, 1987), which has been slower in recent years. How serious any of these factors will be in the long run is still debatable, but theoretical concerns and empirical evidence highlight the potential negative effect of payment reform on patient care.

Recent payment reforms may also jeopardize the future of clinical education programs. In the past, a large proportion of the cost of graduate medical education and allied health professions education were financed through patient care revenues. Third-party payors, which paid hospitals on a charge or cost basis, enabled hospitals to support clinical education through cross-subsidization. Theoretically, however, as payors become more concerned about the cost of medical care, they may be less willing to pay more to teaching hospitals for patient care than to community hospitals, particularly when patients are being treated for similar conditions. If this is the case, then teaching hospitals will no longer be able to use patient care revenues to cross-subsidize teaching activities. Hospitals may be forced to identify the separate costs associated with clinical education, explore alternative financing arrangements to find continued teaching activities, or eliminate teaching activities altogether.

We know of no empirical evidence that documents the direct effect of payment reform on clinical education programs. In fact, the 1980s have witnessed a slight increase in the number of teaching programs. That medical education programs have been somewhat protected from recent cost containment initiatives may be explained by changes in the Medicare and Medicaid programs in the 1980s, designed explicitly to support teaching hospitals (Iglehart, 1986; Anderson and Lave, 1986). However, if public support for teaching hospitals or clinical education wanes, then the future of clinical education may be uncertain. Recent changes in Medicare reimbursement principles for direct medical education suggest that significant reductions are coming.

Efforts to control the federal deficit and lower the rate of federal spending have slowed the rate of increase in spending for biomedical research and technology development. As a result, academic medical centers, which had grown accustomed to substantial annual increases in support from the National Institutes of Health and other public and private sponsors of clinical research, are beginning to examine their own financial liability for new and existing research projects. In the past, the cost to the hospital of conducting hospital-based clinical research and clinical trials was not a major issue. However, as the economic environment of the hospital changes and as insurers become more reluctant to pay the higher patient care costs associated with clinical research, hospitals may become less willing to cross-subsidize underfunded or unsponsored research.

The decline in spending for biomedical research has been substantial in recent years. Between 1980 and 1986, spending for biomedical research grew at an average annual rate of 3.5 percent—a rate lower than inflation or any other component of the health care sector (Anderson and Erickson, 1987). Hospitals are beginning to be concerned about the cost of conducting clinical research and whether they should receive a portion of the overhead payments, which has traditionally gone only to their medical schools. The New England Medical Center may be on the vanguard in capturing all of the overhead associated with research projects by constructing a research building and hiring researchers directly (Anderson and Russe, 1987). Other academic medical centers are also trying to capture some of the revenues associated with clinical research. This could affect the nature of biomedical research conducted in the United States in a way that may not be in accordance with the public interest.

Changes in hospital financing may also exacerbate problems experienced by the uninsured and the related problems of uncompensated care. Payment reform constrains the ability of hospitals to charge their paying patients rates that allow them to subsidize the cost of uncompensated care. Hospitals that continue to care for uninsured patients are much more likely than others to incur operating losses. In addition, the uninsured population may find it increasingly difficult to get medically necessary treatment.

There is some evidence that hospitals are responding to payment reform by changing their policies concerning care for the poor, so that access to care by the poor is limited. Some hospitals have reduced their emergency rooms hours where the uninsured are most likely to be admitted for treatment (Sloan, Valvona, and Mullner, 1986). Other studies have documented increases in medically inappropriate transfers of uninsured patients (Schiff et al., 1986). Hospitals that have shown an increase in their uncompensated care burden have not raised prices commensurate with the increased cost of providing care to these patients (Hadley and Feder, 1985).

However fragmentary, the data provide a basis for concern about the consequences of payment reform on the future provision of services. At the same time, it must be remembered that payment reforms were designed and implemented to bring about change. It is, therefore, important to evaluate whether these changes are in the public interest. For example, recent payment reforms have no doubt contributed to hospital closings; yet, in an industry characterized by excess capacity, this may not be undesirable. The slowdown of the diffusion of medical technologies may or may not be a matter of social concern. Subsidizing the training of physicians in a period of perceived physician surplus may not be desirable. Under the financing schemes that persisted in the 1970s, policy analysts argued that financial incentives contributed to an excessive diffusion of medical technologies.

With increasing tighter controls on hospital payments, these services. which were traditionally funded through cross-subsidies, have been placed in the public spotlight. In the past, there was little interest in either the cost of these services or their distribution. With the advent of payment reform, the cost of these services and who should pay for them are becoming major policy concerns. The potential public and private payors of these services want more information about their cost, their method of financing, and how they are distributed across payors and hospitals. What hospital administrators, physicians, policy makers, and the general public are beginning to realize is that there is no such thing as a free lunch and that someone must pay for these services if they are going to be provided in the future.

The Organization of the Book

This book is divided into three parts. In the first part (chapters 1 and 2), we examine hospitals, emphasizing the teaching hospital. We begin the discussion with the hospital because this is where the four services are provided. We discuss why teaching hospitals tend to be more costly than other hospitals, identify factors contributing to their relatively higher costs, and present the empirical estimates showing the relative importance of each factor. We also examine the complex ways hospitals are financed, again concentrating on teaching hospitals, because they provide the majority of clinical education, biomedical research, and care for patients requiring complex services. Many of these same hospitals also shoulder a disproportionate share of the care of low-income and uninsured patients.

In the second part (chapters 3 through 6), we move beyond the hospital to the services themselves and focus on them for the remainder of the book. First we review the historical development of each of the four services and then focus on (1) the distribution of each service across hospitals; (2) the cost of the service; (3) the current method of financing the service; (4) the method of controlling the scope and level of services provided.

In the distribution section, we evaluate the extent to which each service is concentrated in a small number of institutions, exploring, for example, the uneven geographic distribution of certain hospital services and the effect of uneven distribution on access. Determining the cost of a service has become increasingly important as insurers, government policy makers, and hospital administrators continue to identify the activities they are willing to pay for. We then describe current financing arrangements for each of the services. Because none are entirely self-supporting, hospitals have developed an elaborate system of cross-subsidization to pay for them. To understand the potential consequences of payment reform and cost containment initiatives, it is useful to understand the financial arrangements that support each service.

We then examine the ways in which the government, payors, and providers exercise control over the provision of these unfunded or underfunded services. In most other industries, the financing and control of services are linked. Typically, whoever pays for a good exercises some control over what will be produced and how it will be produced. However, this is not generally the case in the hospital sector. In the past, government and other third-party payors did not exert much control over the delivery of services, leaving most of the control to the hospitals and professional associations. If the balance of control shifts from providers to the government and insurers, the production and distribution of these services is likely to be affected.

The third part of the book, chapters 7 through 10, presents policy options. For each service, a specific proposal is developed that considers the cost of production, alternative funding sources, the implications for the distribution of services, and the balance between public and private control.

In chapter 7, we present specific proposals for modifying hospital payment systems to account for differences in the cost of providing patient care. Special attention is given to modifications that will improve the access to care and the quality of care for patients requiring complex services. A fundamental reform of the graduate medical education system is proposed in chapter 8, which would substantially change the locus of responsibility for the support of this education from the insurer to the hospital, the faculty practice plan, and the resident.

The proposal in chapter 9 for changing the system of paying for biomedical research is less comprehensive because of a lack of basic information about the current system. Instead, we propose several areas for future research and data collection so that a financing policy can be developed to support hospital-based clinical research and technology development.

In chapter 10, we propose that the tax deduction of employer-provided health care coverage be altered to encourage the uninsured to purchase health insurance. In addition, a system of federal and state subsidies is proposed to help low-income uninsured persons obtain health insurance.

part I | Teaching Hospitals

For most of this book, we discuss four services: complex patient care, clinical education, biomedical research, and uncompensated care. We begin, however, by examining the hospital, because it is where many of these services are provided.

In chapter 1 we examine why certain hospitals have higher costs than other hospitals. The chapter begins with a detailed review of the factors influencing hospital costs. It then discusses what costs should be considered when making cost comparisons and how to estimate these costs. Particular attention should be given to the summary of the empirical results, since they form the basis for the policy recommendations spelled out later. We explore the methods of financing hospital services in chapter 2. This chapter begins with a discussion of the sources of hospital revenues, with a particular emphasis on patient care revenues, since they represent the bulk of hospital revenues. It then discusses how revenue sources vary by type of hospital and how they have changed over time. The final section of chapter 2 discusses the flow of funds within the academic medical center.

Chapters 1 and 2 center on the hospital for several reasons. Many of these services are produced primarily in hospitals, and traditionally they have been financed through cross-subsidies. As a result, the future provision of these services may depend upon the financial viability of certain institutions. Second, because these services are often provided jointly, the allocation of costs to specific activities is somewhat arbitrary. Third, these services are disproportionately produced in a small number of hospitals. Thus, policies that affect these hospitals indirectly affect the provision of these services.

Any discussion of the hospital must recognize that hospitals are not homogeneous. For this reason, we have developed a simple hospital typology, similar to that used by many other researchers (Sloan, Feldman, and Steinwald, 1983). Although other studies have used different methods to group hospitals, the results are generally similar.

We classified hospitals into four groups. To create the first two groups, we used criteria developed by the Association of American Medical Colleges (AAMC). Members of the Council of Teaching Hospitals (COTH) are separated into two groups, depending on ownership status and degree of interaction between the hospital and a medical school. The first group, major COTH, consists of 119 hospitals that are members of the Council of Teaching Hospitals and either are owned and operated by the university that operates the medical school or have significant overlap between the medical school department chairmen and the clinical chiefs of staff. Minor COTH, the second group, consists of 210 hospitals that are members of the Council of Teaching Hospitals but do not meet either of the two other requirements.

None of the hospitals in groups three and four are members of COTH. Group three, other teaching, has residency programs approved by the American Medical Association (AMA) or spent at least $15,000 on residency programs in 1986. The use of AMA-approved residencies as the only criterion would have classified some hospitals with large financial commitments to residency programs as nonteaching hospitals. The requirement that a minimum of $15,000 be spent to be classified as a teaching hospital was necessary to ensure that a minimum level of graduate medical education was provided at the hospital during the year. Finally, the last group is nonteaching hospitals. A few of the hospitals that fall into this category have residents, but their programs are not AMA approved, and they spend less than $15,000 on educational programs.

In 1986, 5,542 institutions were identified as short-term general community hospitals. The remaining hospitals were either long-term hospitals (hospitals with an average patient stay of over thirty days) or federal hospitals. Table I-1 presents summary data on community hospitals according to the hospital categories used in this book. Approximately 80 percent are nonteaching institutions, while only 5.9 percent are members of COTH. However, on average, COTH hospitals are significantly larger than other hospitals, and consequently their beds make up about 20 percent of the total bed supply. However, the size of the standard deviation of the number of beds in each group is a reminder that the hospitals in each category are dramatically different in terms of size.

On average, however, the capacity of each group of hospitals to diagnose and treat patients with complex medical conditions is quite different. For example, more than 25 percent of COTH hospitals have on-site lithotripters, which allow for the noninvasive removal of kidney

Table I-1.   Selected Characteristics of Short-Term Community Hospitals, 1986

Characteristic	Major COTH	Minor COTH	Other Teaching	Nonteaching	All Hospitals
Hospitals					
Number	119	210	859	4,354	5,542
Percent	2.15	3.79	15.50	78.56	100.0
Beds					
Average number in hospital	615	560	307	116	173
(Standard deviation)	(282)	(223)	(160)	(95)	(173)
Total number	73,208	117,619	263,438	505,236	959,501
Percent	7.63	12.26	27.46	52.66	100
Dollar expenditure per discharge	5,432	4,557	3,614	2,419	3,022

Source: Based on data from American Hospital Association, A, 1986.

stones by using shock waves (see table 3-3); only 1 percent of non-teaching hospitals have this state-of-the-art technology. Open heart surgery is representative of the complex, very technological surgical procedures that take place in hospitals today. Nearly 90 percent of major COTH hospitals have open-heart surgical facilities, compared to 3 percent of nonteaching hospitals.

The primary source of payment for patient care services also varies by type of hospital (see table 2-3). Compared to other groups of hospitals, major COTH hospitals have a higher proportion of patients without insurance and of Medicaid patients and a smaller percentage of patients covered by commercial insurance policies. In general, revenues that a hospital receives for providing care to uninsured and Medicaid patients do not cover the full cost of treating them, while the revenues received from commercial insurance companies usually exceed the full cost of care. Consequently, the financial environment varies systematically across the different groups of hospitals.

Not surprisingly, since the typology is partially based on a hospital's commitment to clinical education, the amount of training that takes place in hospitals differs significantly across the four categories. Major COTH hospitals train over 45 percent of all residents in the United States (see table 4-5). The importance of residency training in these hospitals is underscored by the fact that there are on average approximately 0.38 residents per hospital bed. Minor COTH hospitals train over 33 percent of all residents. The involvement in graduate medical education is much lower in minor COTH hospitals, which train only 0.17 residents per bed. Minor teaching hospitals train about

20 percent of residents. However, for these institutions, training is only a minor activity, with 0.04 residents per bed.

On average, hospital cost per discharge and hospital cost per day vary significantly across the groups of hospitals. The cost per discharge is more than 100 percent higher in major COTH hospitals than in nonteaching hospitals. In 1986, the average cost per discharge varied from $5,432 in major COTH hospitals to $2,419 in nonteaching hospitals (see table I-1). While a simple comparison of costs per discharge does not consider the multitude of factors that could explain the variation in costs, the magnitude of the variations suggest that teaching hospitals may be at a comparative disadvantage in a price-competitive environment if the services that add to this higher cost are not financed explicitly.

Although the data included throughout the book indicate that, on average, hospitals within each group vary along important dimensions, they conceal the heterogeneity among hospitals within a group. At times it is useful to disaggregate the groups even further. This is particularly true when we consider the treatment of patients without health insurance. In this case, it is the public hospitals that assume the greater role of treating this population (Commonwealth Task Force on Academic Medical Centers, 1985). With the exception of the commitment to graduate medical education, as measured by the number of residents per bed, there is considerable overlap between the categories. For instance, some hospitals in the minor COTH group and even the minor teaching group may admit patients with more complicated medical conditions than those in the major COTH hospitals. Bad debt and charity patients may represent a higher proportion of inpatient load in a minor teaching hospital than in a major COTH hospital. Thus, in some of the discussion to follow, we may find the typology is not useful in certain areas, because the amount of variation within each group is so large.

chapter 1 | Hospital Costs

The costs of providing services in hospitals vary considerably. In 1986, for example, the costs per hospital discharge in each of the four groups of hospitals ranged from $2,419 in nonteaching hospitals to $5,432 in major COTH hospitals. However, because of the considerable variation among hospitals with respect to the types of patients treated, scope of services provided, and geographic location, these simple cost comparisons can be very misleading indicators of their relative cost. In addition, if we look at only costs per discharge, we ignore many of the other services (such as clinical education) provided by hospitals.

There have been innumerable investigations into the reasons why costs vary across hospitals. Most early studies were concerned with health planning issues. A typical question asked was whether there is a most efficient-sized hospital, which should be encouraged through the planning process. Although attention given to health planning has waned, that given to understanding variation in costs has not.

Policy issues have changed over time. The current focus reflects the extent to which Medicare and some Medicaid programs have implemented prospective payment systems or other forms of hospital rate setting. Policy makers need to understand why costs vary across hospitals to (1) make judgments about which factors to take into consideration in setting rates and (2) be aware of the implications of not taking certain factors into account. For example, if there is a hospital characteristic that is related to hospital costs but is not taken into consideration when setting rates, then hospitals with that characteristic will be disadvantaged financially. Researchers, however, are interested in using cost analyses not only to feed information into the policy process but also to evaluate the outcomes of that process. In addition, an examination of why certain hospitals are more expensive than others will provide insight into how specific types of hospitals will fare in a price competitive world.

Factors Influencing Hospital Costs

The most important factor influencing hospital costs is the levels of the hospital's output: the types and volumes of patient care provided (both inpatient and outpatient), the hospital's teaching commitment, and the extent of research undertaken. The costs of producing each of these services vary, depending on the quality and scope of the services, the prices the hospital pays for their factors of production (i.e., nurses, drugs, food, diagnostic equipment, etc.), and the efficiency with which they are produced. All of these factors, which are discussed in greater detail below, vary across hospitals and lead to differences in their costs. Uncompensated care is not listed as a factor affecting the level of hospital costs. Unlike the other services, uncompensated care is defined by the absence of revenue for services provided and not as a generator of costs.

Patient Care

The total costs incurred by a hospital depend upon the number and types of patients seen in the inpatient setting, in the outpatient department, and in the emergency room. More resources are needed in the emergency room to care for a trauma patient than for a patient with a respiratory problem who has failed to see a physician and has become worried. More inpatient resources are needed to treat a patient who has had a coronary bypass than one who has had a cholecystectomy. Even for patients with the same diagnosis, more resources are likely to be needed to treat those who are more critically ill or who have more complications and comorbidities.

Characteristics of the patient other than clinical condition also may affect the cost of treatment and, consequently, hospital costs. For example, patients who are admitted through emergency rooms are less likely to have a regular doctor, and more resources may be required to establish their diagnoses. Low-income patients clinically similar to other patients may be kept longer in the hospital because their home environments may be less conducive to convalescence. In addition, hospitals that treat a large number of low-income patients may incur higher costs in responding to the special needs of these patients by providing additional services, such as social work and patient education.

Because the cost of care varies with the nature and type of patients seen, measures describing the patient population must be included in any study of hospital costs. There has been extensive work in the development of hospital case mix measures (for a general review see Lave and Lave, 1984; Hornbrook, 1982; Jencks and Dobson, 1987). Case mix measurement continues to be the subject of very active research.

To measure case mix, surrogate measures, such as scope of services, were used initially as proxies for the differences in case mixes across hospitals. These measures are inherently unsatisfactory for three reasons. First, while case mix varies with scope of services, a listing of the facilities offered is not a sensitive measure of the patient population. For example, two hospitals, each of which has an open-heart surgical suite, would have quite different patient populations if the suite were used once a month in one hospital and once a day in the other. Second, scope of services is a measure of the inputs used by the hospital to produce patient care rather than a measure of output of patient care. Economists and other researchers would rather use output measures, because they indicate what the hospital is actually providing rather than what it has the capability of providing. Third, when policy makers began to look for methods to set hospital payment rates in a way that considered case mix, there was fear that using scope of services as a proxy for case mix would lead to an increase in services offered and to a duplication of facilities in a community.

Once computer files listing the age, sex, race, diagnoses, and procedures for all hospital discharges became available, it was possible to develop better measures of a hospital's inpatient population. For the first time, the output of the hospital could be measured in terms of the types of patients treated rather than the nature of services provided. At present, the most widely used patient classification system is the diagnosis-related group, or DRG (Fetter, 1982). Data on the characteristics of patients (diagnosis, procedure, discharge status, and age) are used to classify them into DRGs.

The DRGs can be used to compare the costs of treating individual patients; or data on all patients can be combined to create a case mix index for the hospital. The case mix index is created by assigning a cost or charge weight to each DRG and multiplying the proportion of the hospital's patients in each DRG by the weight of the DRG. This index is an estimate of the relative costliness of the hospital's case mix compared to that of the average hospital. For instance, a hospital with a DRG case mix index of 1.2 is assumed to have an inpatient population that is 20 percent more costly to treat than that of the average hospital (Pettingill and Vertrees, 1982).

Although the DRG case mix index has been widely used to measure the costliness of a hospital's inpatient population, critics claim that DRG groupings are not homogeneous and that, therefore, the index may be a misleading indicator of the relative costliness of a given hospital's inpatient caseload. Some analysts have suggested that other patient classification systems, such as the severity-of-illness index (Horn, Horn, and Sharkey, 1984; Horn et al., 1986), disease staging (Gonnella, Hornbrook, and Lewis, 1984) and MEDISGRPS (Brewster et al., 1985) be used to supplement the DRGs; while other analysts have proposed that classification systems such as the patient management categories (Young et al., 1983) should replace the DRGs. Unfortunately, few studies have compared these different systems (Berman et al., 1986). HCFA has funded a team of Canadian researchers to conduct a large-scale systematic comparison of the different systems, and the results should be available in early 1990.

Researchers have used measures such as the proportion of the hospital's inpatient population covered by Medicaid, the proportion of bad debt and charity patients (Anderson and Lave, 1986) and the proportion of inpatients admitted through the emergency room (Thorpe, 1988b) as proxies for patients who, because of their social status, may need more services. These patients may be sicker upon admission in ways not captured by the DRGs and may be more difficult to discharge because of home conditions. The variables represent characteristics of the inpatient population that make them more costly to treat.

Clinical Education

The establishment and operation of clinical education programs increase hospital costs. Costs associated with clinical education have been classified into two categories, direct and indirect. Direct costs are explicitly associated with the salaries and fringe benefits paid by the teaching program to residents and to attending physicians and other instructors, and for educational supplies and associated overhead costs. Direct costs vary with the size and scope of the teaching programs.

The presence of teaching programs may lead to higher patient care costs due to the active role of residents and academic physicians in the care of these patients; these costs are the indirect costs of graduate medical education. Researchers have put forth several hypotheses to explain why these costs are higher in teaching hospitals:

1. The resident's relative inexperience in the management of patient care and the consequent increased use of ancillary services (Garg et al.; 1982, Schroeder and O'Leary, 1977).
2. The tendency to try to make a more accurate diagnosis both for educational purposes and to satisfy the need to know of the more academically minded physicians, even in those circumstances where treatment may not be modified by the findings (Reuben, 1984).
3. The increased availability of state-of-the-art teaching facilities and treatment technologies.
4. The fact that very sick patients may be treated more aggressively in these institutions (Garber, Fuchs, and Silverman, 1984).
5. Decreased productivity of other employees, such as nurses.

To quantify the effect that clinical education has on hospital costs, it is necessary to measure the extent of clinical education in a particular hospital. Frequently, teaching activity is measured by a set of categorical variables, such as the four categories of hospitals described in the Introduction. Recently, researchers have begun to measure commitment to teaching by the ratio of residents per bed (Pettingill and Vertrees, 1982; Anderson and Lave, 1986; Arthur Young, 1987).

Biomedical Research

Theoretically, research costs, also, can be divided into direct and indirect costs. Direct costs include the costs of personnel (the investigator and staff), computer time, the drugs and equipment being examined, and associated overhead costs. Indirect costs involve the increased patient care costs that may be incurred because there is a research program. Neither direct nor indirect costs of clinical research have been studied extensively, and there are no good proxies for extent of research.

In addition to clinical research, product development also takes place within hospitals. Medical advances such as new cancer therapies, bone marrow transplants, artificial joints and organ transplants, and new diagnostic technologies such as magnetic imaging are generally initiated at academic hospitals before diffusing to other institutions (Russell, 1979). These services may increase hospital costs substantially, especially in the early years of development, when protocols are not well established, tests are often repeated, and the new technologies are used in conjunction with those they will eventually replace (Anderson and Steinberg, 1984a).

Quality of Care

The costs of providing hospital services should vary with the quality of services rendered. Most of the work on quality in hospitals has focused on the quality of inpatient services provided. Patient care services are often classified into two groups: amenities, as reflected in the quality of the food, the pleasantness of the environment, and so forth—the so-called hotel functions; and technical care, as reflected in the medical management of the patient. Most attention has been directed to the latter category.

The concept of the quality of care has proven to be quite elusive. While there is no universally accepted definition of quality, there is general agreement among experts that it is a multidimensional construct with at least three components: structure, process, and outcome (Donabedian, 1980). Although there is often an implicit assumption that improvements in quality will increase the costs of care, this conclusion does not necessarily follow. In fact, costs could either increase or decrease as the quality of care increases. For example, additional nursing hours, which would probably increase costs, could lead to higher quality of care through higher patient satisfaction and improved patient outcomes. Conversely, improvements in quality as represented by decreases in iatrogenic disease, nosocomial infections, and surgical complications would lower hospital costs.

There are few objective indicators of the quality of care at the hospital level. In early cost studies, accreditation by the Joint Committee of Hospitals (JCAH, now the Joint Committee of the Association of Health Care Organizations) was used as a proxy for quality. However, since the overwhelming majority of hospitals were accredited, this was not a discriminating variable. Moreover, to use JCAH accreditation as a proxy for quality is to use structure and process criteria measures. In general, researchers are reluctant to rely on structure and process measures as quality measures, preferring instead to use outcome measures. In addition, since these measures are likely to be associated with more services and hence higher costs, the relationship between quality and cost then becomes tautological.

There has been some recent work on the construction of quality measures. These include hospital mortality rates, hospital readmission rates (Anderson and Steinberg, 1984b) and identification of adverse outcomes (Arthur Young, 1987). With the exception of the Arthur Young studies, these quality measures have not been used in empirical studies of hospital costs. It should be pointed out that the development of methods to measure hospital quality are high on the agenda of both the Joint Committee of the Association of Health Care Organizations and the Health Care Financing Administration (HCFA).

Input Prices

The cost of producing hospital services depends upon the prices that hospitals pay for the inputs they use to produce those services. The prices of inputs such as drugs and equipment, which are purchased in national markets, may not vary significantly across institutions or by geographic region. Other inputs, such as electricity and food, are purchased in regional markets, and although their prices may not vary across hospitals within a region, the costs could vary significantly across regions. Finally, most labor services, such as those of secretaries, technicians, and nurses, are purchased in local markets; and hospitals must compete with other firms in their market areas for these factors of production. As a result of the geographic variation in factor prices, the costs of providing hospital services will vary geographically.

Geographic data on factor prices, with the exception of labor, are very scarce. Consequently, factor prices are usually proxied by the cost of labor. Two approaches have been used: one is to calculate the prices paid by a specific hospital for labor, the other is to use the average prices paid for hospital labor in the geographic area in which the hospital is located.

Economies of Scale and Scope

The cost of producing hospital services also depends upon the nature of the underlying technology. The two dimensions of technology of primary interest are economy of scale and economy of scope. Economies of scale are related to the relationship between unit costs (cost per discharge) and the volume of output (number of discharges). If there are no economies of scale, then unit costs do not vary with changes in the level of output; if there are economies of scale, then unit costs fall as output increases; and conversely, if there are diseconomies of scale, unit cost rise as output increases. The scale of operation is usually measured either by the number of beds operated by a hospital or the number of patient discharges (days).

Economies of scope indicate whether it is more efficient to render patient care to a wide variety of patients at a single hospital or to have hospitals specialize in the treatment of certain cases. An economy of scope is usually measured by the number of facilities and services offered. If there are economies of scope, it will cost less to provide care to two different types of patients in one facility rather than to have them taken care of in hospitals that specialize in the treatment needed by each of these patients.

The nature of economies of scale and scope will influence the structure of the health care system. For example, if there are economies of scale, then small institutions will have a difficult time surviving in a competitive environment. If there are economies of scope, hospitals in a competitive environment will begin to specialize in the treatment of specific kinds of cases.

Standby Costs

Some hospitals incur costs by providing services that are used infrequently or on an emergency basis but that must be staffed continuously. These services are often called standby services. As Cowing, Holtman, and Powers (1983) explained, "if one views the hospital in addition to providing direct or anticipated patient care as also providing sufficient capacity to assure that hospitals are available should an individual need care, this insurance or option demand should be treated as yet another service by the hospital" (p. 373).

The concept of standby services has been difficult to quantify. Some analysts have considered measures based on the hospital's occupancy rate as indicators of standby capacity (Joskow, 1980). Still others have looked at whether the presence of certain specific services, such as burn units or helicopter rescue services, have a significant effect on costs once other factors have been taken into account (Commonwealth Task Force on Academic Medical Centers, 1985).

Technical Efficiency

The level of hospital costs will depend on how efficient hospitals are in treating different types of patients. Technical efficiency can vary across hospitals either because the various departments of the hospitals are managed differently or because physicians have different practice patterns. Physicians differ in how they manage the treatment of patients with respect to test ordering, therapies and drugs prescribed, and length of hospital stay. These differences give rise to differences in the observed costs of different hospitals. A number of factors can affect technical efficiency, including hospital ownership and control, payor mix, regulatory environment, and economic environment.

Hospital Ownership and Control   Some hospitals are independent, freestanding institutions, while others are part of large chains in which many of the decisions with respect to capital, staffing, and purchasing are made centrally. Some hospitals are nonprofit institutions, some are public institutions, and others are strictly for-profit institutions. The hospital's decision-making environment varies by type of ownership and organization. For example, managers of public hospitals may have to follow civil service rules in hiring employees or may be required to purchase services from approved suppliers. Managers of other institutions may have fewer restrictions on their decisions: managers of for-profit institutions are more likely to be rewarded on the basis of their institution's profits, while managers of nonprofit hospitals may be rewarded according to other criteria, such as their ability to introduce state-of-the-art technology to their community. These differences in the nature of the hospital's ownership may have an independent effect on the cost of providing services.

The Hospital's Payor Mix   Payor mix varies across hospitals. In some hospitals, the majority of patients are covered by insurance policies, which pay hospitals on the basis of retrospective costs or posted charges. In other hospitals, the majority of patients are self-paying or are covered by indemnity policies, which pay only a fixed amount per day. And in still other hospitals, most of the revenues come in the form of prospectively set payments. Incentives differ across these institutions. In hospitals that receive most of their revenues from cost-based or charge-based payment systems, there is less financial pressure to produce efficiently, more room for managerial slack, and less pressure to be concerned about whether the benefit to be gained from doing more for the patient is worth the cost. In hospitals that receive most of their revenues from prospective payment systems, there are stronger economic incentives to produce care efficiently. Thus, differences in payor mix among hospitals may be associated with differences in their costs.

The Regulatory Environment   The laws and regulations governing payment for hospital services and the nature of external constraints on hospital decision makers vary considerably in the United States. For example, hospitals located in states that are subject to rate control may have stronger incentives to contain costs than hospitals in other states. Administrators of hospitals located in areas with certificate-of-need programs may have less freedom in making capital purchases. This restriction on the actions of hospital decision makers could have an effect on the cost of care provided.

The Competitive Environment   The nature and the extent of hospital competition may influence costs. Hospitals could compete for patients either on the basis of price, which should be associated with lower costs, or on the basis of services, which would increase costs.

Other Factors

A number of other factors, more difficult to classify, will affect the cost and quality of patient care provided by different hospitals. For example, the availability of resources such as home health services, nursing homes, and intermediate care facilities varies across regions. Consequently, some hospitals may be able to discharge patients to lower levels of care, while other hospitals may have to keep patients in the hospital until they are ready to go home. Other things being equal, the cost of hospital care per discharge should be lower in the former case. In addition, the per capita income of the county in which the hospital is located may influence hospital costs. If people with higher incomes demand more services, then this will be reflected in the cost of care. Other demographic and income variables may have similar effects.

Before turning to methods of estimating the importance of these various factors in influencing hospital cost, we should stress that many of the factors discussed above are hypothesized to influence costs through their effect on the quantity and nature of services provided and not through their effect on the types of patient treated. We have classified these factors as those that influence the technical efficiency with which care is provided. This label is a bit misleading. These factors may influence the quality of care provided in ways that we value but that we cannot measure. However, without empirical measures of quality, we cannot unambiguously assign these increased costs to technical inefficiency or to increased quality.

Developing a Cost Function

One approach to examining the relationship between costs and other variables is to estimate a cost function. Essentially, a general cost function repeats the earlier discussion in mathematical terms and can be specified as in the equation below, where hospital costs (*HC*) are a function of outputs (*O*), quality (*Q*), scope of services (*SCP*), scale of services (*SCL*), factor prices (*P*) and efficiency (*E*):

$$HC = f(O, Q, SCP, SCL, P, E).$$

A cost function is estimated by the use of a multivariate statistical technique called regression analysis. In this technique, the dependent variable, cost, is regressed against the independent variables (*O*, *Q*, *SCP*, *SCL*, *P*, *E*), and the influence of each independent variable on the dependent variable is determined. In estimating a particular equation, the analyst must (1) identify the types of costs of interest (total, per day, per discharge, hospital only, or hospital and physician), (2) identify the unit of measurement (hospital or discharge), and (3) specify both the independent variables and the functional form. Many of these issues are very technical and need not concern us here. (See Cowing, Holtman, and Powers, 1983; Lave and Lave, 1984; Breyer, 1987, for a more detailed discussion.) However, some of these are quite important; and understanding the issues facilitates a general understanding of some of the public policy debates that surround hospital costs.

Which Costs?

Conceptually, one can focus on one of two general types of costs in comparing the costs of different hospitals. One is the costs incurred by the hospital in providing hospital services (hospital services); the other is the cost of taking care of patients in hospitals, which include the costs of both the hospital and physician services (full hospital costs). There is no strict boundary between hospital and physician costs, since each provides some services that are substitutes for those provided by the other.

The general point can be clarified if one considers the costs of teaching hospitals vis-à-vis those of other hospitals. The salaries of interns and residents are recorded as hospital costs. However, this staff provides services that substitute for those provided by fee-for-service physicians. As a consequence, compared to other hospitals, hospital costs may be higher in teaching hospitals, but the full cost of hospitalization may not be.

With the exception of certain hospitals, such as those operated by the Veterans Administration, most physicians are not salaried, and hospitals have no records of the costs of physician services rendered. Consequently, to study the full costs of hospitalization, analysts have to either painstakingly build up a physician use-and-charge profile through the examination of medical records or assemble special data bases by merging both hospital and physician claims records. This is very difficult to do, as physicians' and hospitals' claims are often paid by separate insurance companies, which use different patient identification numbers. Even if the claims are paid by the same insurance companies, they may not keep the physicians' and hospitals' claims together. As a result, in most studies of hospital cost functions, hospital costs rather than full costs are the focus.

Total Cost or Inpatient Costs?

With few exceptions (Grannemann, Brown, and Pauly, 1986), most analysts have investigated factors related to inpatient costs per day or per admission rather than total hospital costs. In this case, some adjustment must be made for the costs attributable to other hospital activities, such as outpatient services, emergency room services, research, and clinical education, which vary from hospital to hospital. Since all hospital products use some of the same hospital resources (e.g., administrative overhead and laboratory services) and some services are produced simultaneously (the training of residents and the rendering of patient care), the allocation of costs to the different activities is somewhat arbitrary. However, accounting and other conventions that allocate expenses among the various activities have been developed and are used by most analysts.

In addition to using standard conventions for determining inpatient costs, most analysts have excluded the direct costs of graduate education from total hospital costs before examining cost variation across hospitals. Including these costs in the hospital's cost base would inflate the cost of patient care in teaching hospitals relative to nonteaching hospitals. However, if full costs are used as the dependent variable, then direct costs are included in the costs of teaching hospitals, and an estimate must be made of the cost of services provided by the fee-for-service physician in both sets of hospitals.

The Unit of Analysis

The final issue concerning the dependent variable has to do with the unit of analysis. Most studies examine the variation in costs per discharge or per day at the hospital level. The cost measure is calculated by taking total hospital costs (excluding the direct costs of graduate medical education) allocated to the inpatient sector and dividing them by the number of either hospital discharges or inpatient days. An alternative is to divide total costs by the number of either adjusted admissions or adjusted patient days. In this case, the number of admissions is adjusted upward to account for outpatient activity.

An alternative is to use patient costs as the dependent variable. In this case, a cost per discharge is calculated for each patient. Since no hospital records the costs at the individual patient level, this step involves a number of complex calculations and is an area of active research.

These two measures complement each other. Information may be gained from the analysis of one measure that is not provided by the other. For example, suppose that, controlling for DRGs, there is very little difference in average patient complexity across hospitals; then differences in patient complexity will not account for any of the differences in costs across these hospitals. However, suppose that it costs more to treat a patient with higher complexity; then analyses of patient cost will provide an estimate of the increased costs associated with increase in complexity. Only through patient-level models will a precise estimate of the incremental costs associated with patient severity be available.

Independent Variables

In estimating hospital cost functions, it is important to specify the model as completely as possible, otherwise some of the calculations will be incorrect. In all cost functions, the estimated coefficient of each of the variables is dependent upon the other variables in the model. (The estimated coefficient for a given variable is the quantitative estimate of how that variable influences costs.) Suppose for example that Medicare operating costs, residents per bed, and number of beds are all correlated. Then, if number of beds is excluded from the variables in a cost function analyses of Medicare operating costs per case, then some of the effect of number of beds on costs will be attributed to the number of residents per bed (Anderson and Lave, 1986; Thorpe, 1988a). Excluding the number of beds from this regression would lead to a biased estimate of the effect on costs of residents per bed. Statistically, this is known as omitted variable bias (Pindyck and Rubinfeld, 1981).

However, analysts sometimes intentionally exclude some of the variables known to influence costs. A case in point is the estimation of cost functions that includes only those variables used to adjust for payments under prospective payment systems. In this case, the coefficient of each variable indicates how the payment should vary with each hospital characteristic, if it is decided that hospitals with that characteristic should not be differentially impacted by the payment system. When comparing results of different models, it is important to know which variables were included in the model and why.

The Structure of the Model

Finally, analysts must specify the nature of the functional relationship between costs and the dependent variables they want to investigate. The issue of appropriate specification is very technical. Theoretically, the form of the cost function should be based on assumptions about the underlying production process, and although some analysts have attempted to derive such functions (Cowing, Holtman, and Powers, 1983; Breyer, 1987), most have not. The majority of investigators have analyzed the relationship between the dependent variable (cost per discharge) and the independent variables in a reasonably straightforward fashion by regressing the dependent variable on the independent variables. The most common formulation is a log-log one; this model assumes that variables act in a multiplicative way and is based upon economists' derivation of a production function (Cobb-Douglas production function).

Cost Function Results

Numerous studies of hospital cost functions have been reported (Lave and Lave, 1984; Cowing, Holtman, and Powers, 1983). These studies represent a significant evolution in estimation technique and measurement and in basic understanding of the hospital industry. When estimating cost functions, analysts have used data from different years, different cost measures, and different samples of hospitals. Despite these differences, a general set of conclusions emerges.

Hospital Costs per Case

Table 1-1 provides summary descriptive information on four recent studies that estimated hospital cost functions. We selected these studies to indicate the diversity in the literature. Each used explicit case mix measures and cost data. The main findings of these and other studies are given below.

Case Mix   The average cost per hospital admission depended strongly on the types of patients treated by the hospitals. An increase in a hospital's case mix index was associated with a proportional increase in the hospital's costs. The proxy measures used as surrogates for a sicker patient population, such as percentage of patients on Medicaid, percentage coming in through the emergency room, and percentage of uncompensated care, provided a positive association with costs in most but not all of the studies.

Graduate Medical Education   After adjustment for direct costs of graduate medical education, the costs of teaching hospitals were found to be higher than those of nonteaching hospitals. Costs increased with the commitment to graduate medical education; for example, Sloan, Feldman, and Steinwald (1983) found that the costs of COTH hospitals (their highest classification) were 13 percent higher than those of nonteaching hospitals. Anderson and Lave (1986) found that a 10 percent increase in the number of residents per bed was accompanied by about a 4.6 percent increase in the Medicare operating cost per case. Since the average major COTH hospital has a ratio of .33 residents per bed, these results indicate that, on average, the major COTH hospitals' costs were 14 percent higher than those of nonteaching hospitals, a finding almost identical to that of Sloan, Feldman, and Steinwald. The estimated effect of graduate medical education on costs is very sensitive to model specification.

Factor Prices   All of the studies showed higher hospital costs in areas that paid a higher price for labor. Unionization also leads to an increase in hospital costs per discharge (Salkever, Steinwachs, and Rapp, 1985).

Economies of Scale and Scope   The estimated effect of number of beds on hospital costs varied across studies. Some studies found costs per discharge declined as the size of the hospital increased to about 100 beds, were constant from 100 to 300 beds, and increased above 300 beds. Others found no strong relationship between costs per case and number of beds (Sloan, Feldman, and Steinwald, 1983), while still others found that costs rose steadily (Anderson and Lave, 1986). The range of findings can be explained by the differences in

Table 1-1.   Selected Characteristics of Hospital Cost Functions

Item	Study 1	Study 2
Dependent variable	Average cost per case	Medicare operating cost per discharge
Data	785 U.S. hospitals (nonrandom)	5,216 hospitals
Year	1974, 1977	1981
Patient characteristics	Resource need index (similar to DRG case mix)	Medicare DRG case mix index
Low-income patients	(not included)	Medicaid and no-pay (percent)
Factor prices	Nonphysician personnel divided by number of full-time personnel	Medicare wage index
Teaching specification	Dummy variable representing scope of teaching	Residents per bed
Size	Beds	Beds
Other hospital variables	Distribution of patients by insurance	(not included)
Geographic variables	Regional dummies; per capita income	Size of MSA 6 categories; hospital located in central city

Sources: Study 1, Sloan, Feldman, and Steinwald, 1983; Study 2, Anderson and Lave, 1986; Study 3, Thorpe, 1988a; Study 4, Lewin and Associates, 1986.
Note: Hospitals with incomplete information were excluded.

the way the size variable was specified and by the fact that the coefficient of beds was sensitive to other variables included in the model.

Standby Costs   Analysts have not made much progress in measuring standby costs; consequently, research findings are not very useful. Variables that have been used to proxy standby costs, such as the number of expensive technologies, had a very small effect on costs (Commonwealth Task Force, 1985).

Geographic Variables   Hospital costs varied across the major regions of the country. Other things equal, hospital costs per discharge were lowest in the South and highest in the West. Costs were higher in urban areas than in rural areas (Pettingill and Vertrees, 1982; Cromwell, 1985). Costs rose with the size of the metropolitan statistical area (MSA) in which the hospital was located (Anderson and Lave, 1986). Some studies found that costs are higher in the central county of the MSA than they are in the ring counties (Ashby, 1984; Anderson and Lave, 1986). Some of these higher costs may be due to unmea-

Study 3	Study 4
Operating cost per discharge	Cost per discharge
270 hospitals in 100 large cities	All Wisconsin hospitals
1985	1985
Medicare DRG case mix index	DRG case mix index
Medicaid, uncompensated care, and ER admittance (percent)	(not included)
Hospital-specific wage index	Medicare wage index
Residents per bed	Residents per bed and teaching categories
Beds	Beds
Proportion covered by Medicare occupancy rate; degree of competition	Scope of services
Regional dummies	(not included)

sured differences in factor prices, some to the fact that the hospitals in larger areas and in central cities have to spend more for services such as security, and some to differences in practice patterns.

Technical Efficiency

In the discussion of the factors affecting hospital costs we used the term technical efficiency to describe factors that were due to differences in the way hospitals were managed or to differences in practice patterns. The effect of many different variables were investigated. Here we focus on three: payor mix, per capita income, and area competition.

Payor Mix   Most analysts have found that payor mix is associated with costs. For example, Sloan, Feldman, and Steinwald (1983) found that the cost per discharge was positively associated with the percentage of the population covered by Medicaid and negatively associated with the proportion of the population covered by commercial insurance. They used payor mix as a surrogate for the hospital's financial environment. They argued that, since most Medicaid programs reimbursed hospitals on the basis of retrospective costs during the period under investigation, as the proportion of Medicaid patients increased, hospital budgets became less constrained. Consequently, it was easier for hospitals to expand the cost base by adding services or by simply being less efficient. On the other hand, as the proportion of patients covered by commercial insurance increased, there were more incentives for providers to use services efficiently both because patients were more sensitive to price if they had to pay deductibles and coinsurance and because efficient hospitals had the potential to earn profits.

However, most analyses of payor mix were conducted before the implementation of the Medicare prospective payment system and the introduction of prospective payment systems by state Medicaid programs. We expect these changes in payment systems will influence the association between costs and percentage of patients covered by the various insurance plans.

Although a number of studies found that hospital costs increased with the percentage of Medicaid admissions, that finding was interpreted differently by various investigators. For example, some investigators assumed that the percentage covered by Medicaid was a surrogate for a more sickly and thus more costly population, while others assumed that it was a surrogate for the hospital's financial environment. Both interpretations are partially true. Only with better patient classification systems will we be able to sort out the relative effects of alternative payment schemes and patient characteristics on hospital costs.

Per Capita Income   Most studies showed that hospital costs increased with the per capita income of the county in which the hospital is located. The most plausible explanation for this finding is that, as incomes rise, people demand more amenities and more services from their hospitals. It is also possible that, since people with higher incomes are more likely to have comprehensive health insurance, hospitals in higher income counties are less financially constrained.

Area Competition   To date, analysts have found that hospital costs were higher in market areas where there were more competing hospitals (Friedman and Shortell, 1988; Robinson and Luft, 1987). These findings are consistent with the argument that hospitals compete for patients by competing for physicians, who bring their patients with them. This competition takes place through the addition of staff and services that make a hospital attractive to physicians. However, we doubt that this effect of competition will be sustained. As payors become aggressive in their search for mechanisms to control their health care costs, it is likely that they will search for hospitals that provide more cost effective care. If hospital costs or prices become an important dimension along which hospitals compete, then we would expect that costs would not be higher, and would perhaps be lower, in those market areas where there are many competing institutions.

Full Costs

Only a few studies analyzed the factors accounting for the variation in the full cost of hospital care across hospitals. The estimated effect of the presence of graduate medical education on hospital costs is likely to be most sensitive to the cost measure used. As noted above, in the studies of hospitals costs, all analysts found that hospital costs (minus the direct costs of graduate medical education) per discharge increased with the number of residents per bed. However, these studies may have overestimated the differences in the cost of providing patient care between teaching and nonteaching hospitals. After all, some of the services provided by residents do substitute for those provided by other physicians; thus it is possible that the full cost of treating patients in teaching hospitals is not as high relative to other hospitals as previous results indicate.

The few studies that looked at full costs found that costs of caring for patients was higher in teaching hospitals but that the cost differential between teaching and nonteaching hospitals was lower. For example, Cameron (1985) compared hospital-only costs and full hospital costs of treating Medicaid patients across different groups of hospitals characterized by their involvement in graduate medical education. He created a data base by merging information on physicians' claims forms, hospital provider forms, and hospital cost reports. The data were adjusted to account for wage differences and case mix differences, as measured by DRGs, across hospitals.

After accounting for wage and case mix differences, the costs in university hospitals (which included residents' salaries) were 33 percent higher than those of nonteaching hospitals. However, when hospital and physician costs were taken into consideration, the differential was reduced to 26 percent. Upon further analysis of the data, Cameron found that residents provided services equal in value to their salaries but that the value of residents' services did not cover any of the so-called indirect costs of clinical education. A second study also found that residents and attending physicians were strong substitutes (Arthur Young, 1986c).

Patient Costs

All of the studies discussed so far used the hospital as the unit of analysis. We now turn to one study that used the patient as the unit of analysis.

Recently, a new data base designed specifically to compare the costs in teaching and nonteaching hospitals has become available. The data contain detailed information on patients' diagnoses, the quality of patient care, clinical education programs, research programs, factor prices, scope of service, and various proxies for technical efficiency. The data were collected from 1983 to 1985 at forty-five hospitals selected from a stratified sample of teaching and nonteaching hospitals. The specific data collection methodology is described elsewhere (Arthur Young, 1986a).

Patient-specific data included the patient's DRG adjusted for severity of illness, whether the patient was on Medicaid, and whether the patient had an adverse event (such as return to surgery or iatrogenic problem).[1] Hospital-specific data included how many of seven costly services the hospital provided (standby costs), the hospital's wage index, the number of residents per bed, the percentage of residency programs on probational accreditation (as a surrogate for the quality of the training programs), the number of fellows (as a surrogate for research programs), the number of other trainees, whether the hospital was a public hospital, and whether the hospital was located in a rate-setting state.[2] Regression results in which the cost per patient was the dependent variable are presented in Table 1-2.

These results indicate that the coefficient of a given variable on

---

1. Patients were classified into DRGs and assigned a severity-of-illness score. For each DRG-severity combination, a cost weight was assigned based on the average cost of treating patients with that combination. Categories with fewer than two observations were dropped from the sample.

2. The seven costly services are (1) an open-heart surgical facility; (2) megavoltage radiation therapy; (3) an organ bank; (4) hemodialysis, inpatient; (5) hemodialysis, outpatient; (6) a genetic counseling department; and (7) a cardiac catheterization laboratory. The index was created by adding the number of services in each hospital.

Table 1-2. Cost Function Analysis of Patient Costs

Factor	Hospital-Only Costs	Hospital and Physician Costs
Constant	7.52	7.99
	(316.4)	(347.4)
Severity of adjusted DRG	.928	.846
	(84.1)	(75.9)
Medicaid	−.065	−.085
	(−3.83)	(−4.45)
Adverse outcomes	.272	.215
	(9.64)	(7.92)
Wage index	.728	.633
	(9.16)	(7.73)
Seven costly services	.067	.157
	(4.99)	(10.99)
Residents per bed	.059	.016
	(9.61)	(2.68)
Probational accreditation (percent)	−.132	−.094
	(−13.96)	(−10.11)
Fellows	.083	.022
	(8.35)	(1.99)
Trainees	−.010	−.015
	(−2.05)	(−2.84)
Public hospital	.062	.139
	(3.07)	(5.97)
Rate setting	−.095	−.142
	(−6.06)	(−8.71)
R^2	.45	.55

Sources: Arthur Young, 1986a, b, c; 1987.
Note: t-statistics in parentheses.

costs depends upon whether one uses the full cost or hospital-only cost. In particular, the estimated coefficient of the ratio of residents to beds decreased in the total cost equation. We interpret this decrease as indicating that the services provided by residents substituted for the services provided by physicians. This finding has major significance for our recommendation presented in chapter 8. Other findings also have relevance to recommendations presented later. For example, the negative coefficient of Medicaid indicates that, controlling for other factors, the Medicaid patient was less costly. In addition, the drop in the size of the coefficient on the Medicaid variable between the hospital cost and total cost suggests that these patients received slightly fewer physician services.

Table 1-3. Hospital Characteristics, by Type of Hospital

Variables	Nonteaching	Major Teaching
	Type of Hospital	
Number of hospitals	4,311	85
Medicare inpatient operating cost per discharge, dollars	1,864.75	4,220.68
Direct teaching costs per discharge, dollars	1.41	316.79
Medicare DRG case mix index	.984	1.186
Medicare wage index	.948	1.121
Medicaid and no-pay patients as a percent of all patients	9.3	15.8
Average number of beds	118.79	634.35
Percent of hospitals in group located in non-SMSA areas	59.5	2.4
Percent of hospitals in group located in SMSAs with 1–2.5 million population	9.7	− 29.1
Percent of hospitals located in SMSAs of over 2.5 million population	9.1	32.9
Percent of urbanized population within county	51.8	87.2

Sources: U.S. Department of Health and Human Services, 1981a, b; Federal Register; American Hospital Association, 1986.

Note: The number of hospitals used in this analysis reflects the number of hospitals for which complete data were available for use in regression analysis. The actual numbers of nonteaching and major teaching hospitals are 4,354 and 119, respectively (see table I-1).

Using Cost Function Analysis to Decompose Costs

In 1981, Medicare operating costs per day were found to be $4,220.68 in major COTH hospitals and $1,864.75 in nonteaching hospitals (Commonwealth Task Force, 1985). These types of hospitals differed substantially, and table 1-3 presents information on their characteristics. A cost function was estimated for all hospitals in the United States, using the model specified by Anderson and Lave (1986) and shown in figure 1-1. The figure shows how the results from these cost functions were used to explain the differences in costs between nonteaching and major teaching hospitals.

The first bar in figure 1-1 shows the mean costs in nonteaching hospitals. The second bar indicates the variables used in the regression model (see table 1-3). The third bar suggests what the regression variables may be measuring. The fourth bar indicates the importance of

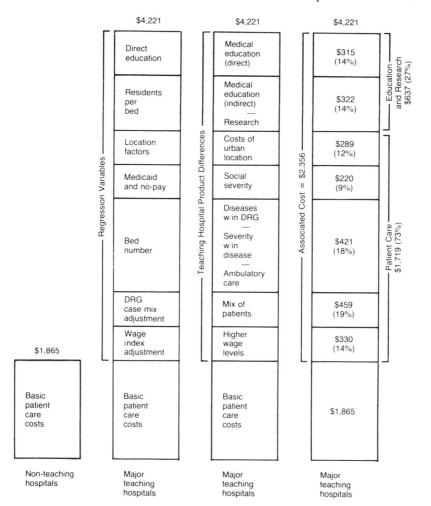

Figure 1-1.   Factors Contributing to Higher Cost per Discharge in Teaching Hospitals, 1981

Sources: U.S. Department of Health and Human Services, 1981b; American Hospital Association, A, 1981; Anderson and Lave, 1986.

Note: Basic patient care costs include standard adjustments for wage level, case mix, service level, and location, reflecting the average cost of production for nonteaching hospitals.

each factor. For example, Medicare operating costs per case are 126 percent higher in major COTH hospitals than in nonteaching hospitals. About 28 percent of this difference is due to the direct and indirect costs of teaching and research, while about 19 percent is due to DRG case mix differences. Approximately 18 percent of the difference is due to the fact that these institutions are larger, and a significant proportion of that difference may be due to unmeasured differences in patient characteristics. Finally, the wages paid in major COTH hospitals are 14 percent higher than those in nonteaching hospitals.

Summary and Conclusion

The costs of providing patient care services vary widely across hospitals. Most of this variation is due to differences in the volumes of services provided, the differences in the kinds of patients treated, the presence and size of graduate medical education programs, and the prices paid for the factors of production. Costs also vary with other characteristics of the hospital (size, payor mix) as well as characteristics of the hospital's environment (competition from other hospitals, regulatory activity, size of the MSA in which it is located, central city location, and region of the country).

Hospital cost function analysis elucidates the reasons why costs vary across hospitals. The results can be used to determine the optimum size of a hospital for planning purposes, to determine the relationship of fixed and variable costs, to assess the cost of an empty bed, to provide guidance to policy makers who are worried about payment policy, to evaluate the effectiveness of past policies, and to examine the consequence of current policy. In chapter 7, we provide some indications of how the results from estimated cost functions can be used to assess the effect of the Medicare prospective payment system and to provide guidance for changing it. In chapter 8, we use the cost function analysis to develop a method of paying for clinical education.

chapter 2 | Financing Hospital Services

The rapid increase in hospital expenditures and the significant variations in costs among hospitals have prompted policy makers, both public and private, to reevaluate what hospital services are provided, how they are provided, and how they are financed. In this chapter we review the financing of hospital services, examine how they have changed, and suggest how they are likely to change further.

Sources of Hospital Revenue

Hospitals derive most of their revenue from patient care. In 1986, gross hospital revenue was approximately $178 billion. Net hospital revenue, which incorporates adjustments for bad debts and discounts and is a more realistic view of hospital receipts, was $148 billion. Net patient care revenue accounted for approximately 93 percent of total net revenue (American Hospital Association, A, 1986).

These proportions have varied over time and across groups of hospitals. As shown in table 2-1, between 1980 and 1984 (the two most recent years for which we can break down these statistics for groups of hospitals), the share of total revenue attributed to patient care increased in both groups of teaching hospitals, while that of nonteaching hospitals was unchanged. On average, teaching hospitals received a higher proportion of their revenue from nonpatient care sources than nonteaching hospitals.

There is only limited information on the breakdown of nonpatient care revenue. Some hospitals, in particular teaching hospitals, receive revenue tied explicitly to the production of specific nonpatient care services, such as biomedical research and clinical education. State appropriations to publicly owned institutions are sometimes shown as nonoperating revenue and sometimes as patient care revenue. In a study that examined the sources of income for university-owned hos-

Table 2-1.   Revenue Source, by Type of Hospital (percent)

Hospital Type	1980 Revenue		1984 Revenue	
	Patient	Nonpatient	Patient	Nonpatient
COTH	85.1	14.9	89.6	10.4
Minor teaching	84.7	15.3	93.0	7.0
Nonteaching	94.1	5.9	93.3	6.7

Source: Based on data from Georgetown University Center for Health Policy.

pitals, the analysts found that about 20.5 percent of the income of state-owned hospitals came from state, city, or county appropriations, whereas only 0.1 percent of the income of privately owned hospitals came from these sources (Association of American Medical Colleges, 1989). The bulk of these appropriations was made to cover the hospitals' deficits (some of which were incurred because the hospitals provided a large volume of uncompensated care), while the rest was tied to the provision of specific services, such as family practice residency programs. Other sources of nonpatient care revenue include income from endowments, community support funds, and operations such as parking garages and gift shops. These sources of revenue tend to be evenly distributed across categories of hospitals.

Given that COTH hospitals produce considerably more nonpatient care services, such as clinical education and biomedical research, than other hospitals, it is somewhat surprising that gross revenue sources are so similar across hospital groups. These data suggest that the cost of producing nonpatient care functions such as teaching are largely cross-subsidized by patient care revenue.

Sources of Patient Revenue

Approximately 90 percent of hospital revenue is derived from third parties; that is, government programs and insurance companies that make payments on behalf of their beneficiaries and enrollees. These third parties have developed multifarious ways to pay hospitals. Unlike most other producers, hospitals receive payments that do not bear a direct relationship to their charges. While a few third-party payors pay hospital charges, the vast majority do not. In some cases, even when the hospital is paid the amount that it charges, a rate-setting commission has constrained its freedom to set these charges. Patients without insurance receive bills based on the hospital's charges, but these patients frequently are unable to pay their bills in full.

In this section, we review the general arrangements under which hospitals receive payments from third parties and how these arrangements have changed (Schwartz, Newhouse, and Williams, 1985; Smith, 1985). We then look at the expected source of patient payment across the four groups of hospitals.

Medicare

When the Medicare program was first implemented, hospitals were reimbursed for "reasonable and necessary" costs they incurred while taking care of Medicare patients, costs that were determined retrospectively (Tierney, 1969). As the program evolved, the formula for calculating reasonable and necessary costs was modified. Congress began placing limitations on how much could be paid.

In 1976, Medicare placed limits on payment for routine (room and board) costs. If a hospital's routine cost per day was significantly above the routine cost of comparable hospitals, the excess cost was not reimbursed, because it was considered unreasonable (Lave, 1985). In 1982, the Tax Equity and Fiscal Responsibility Act (TEFRA) used this same principle but incorporated the DRG classification system to broaden the definition of costs under review. A hospital's costs were considered unreasonable if its case mix adjusted cost per discharge was significantly higher than the cost of comparable hospitals or if the increase in its cost per discharge was above that set by the government.

In 1983, Congress implemented the Medicare prospective payment system (PPS) by amending the Social Security Act. PPS now covers all hospitals and patients with the exception of free-standing psychiatric, rehabilitation, long-term, and children's hospitals as well as discharges from exempted psychiatric and rehabilitation units in general hospitals. Under PPS, payments to hospitals are made in four parts. Payments to cover operating costs for Medicare patients are made through prospectively set DRG payments. Payments to cover capital costs and the direct costs of graduate medical education are made on the basis of costs actually incurred by each hospital; a recent congressional decision bases the capital payment on a percentage of capital costs. Payments for indirect medical education are made through a formula-based adjustment to PPS rates (see chapter 4).

In determining PPS payment rates, all patients are classified into one of 475 DRGs (the number keeps increasing) for the purpose of payment. Each DRG is assigned a charge weight, which reflects the relative cost of treating a patient in that DRG compared to the cost of treating the average Medicare patient.[1] At the same time, a standardized rate is determined for each hospital. This rate is based upon the national average cost of treating a Medicare patient, which is then adjusted to take into consideration factors that cause costs to be higher or lower. Current adjustment factors include the wage rate in the hospital's geographic area, number of residents per bed, and number of Medicaid patients. Separate national average costs per discharge are calculated for urban and rural hospitals.

To determine the payment a hospital receives for taking care of a patient in a given DRG, its standardized rate is multiplied by the relative cost weight for that DRG. Through an outlier adjustment, hospitals receive extra payment for those patients who are significantly more costly than the average patient in that DRG. Outlier payments, by law, are limited to a specific percentage of total DRG payments.

Each year, an explicit decision is made about how much to increase the standardized rate. In theory, this decision is based on the increase in prices that hospitals have to pay for their inputs (the hospital market basket), an allowance for technological change, and an adjustment for productivity changes. However, in practice, the decision has been driven by budgetary consideration. The allowed rates of increase for fiscal years 1984, 1985, 1986, and 1987 were 3.26, 4.15, 0.21, and 1.15 percent, respectively. These rates were significantly lower than the increases in the cost of the hospital's market basket (ProPAC, 1987).

A simple example shows how Medicare payments vary across hospitals, depending on the type of patients discharged. Suppose that patients can be grouped into one of only three DRGs: DRG 90 (simple pneumonia and pleurisy, patients aged eighteen to sixty-nine), DRG 121 (circulatory diseases with acute myocardial infarction), and DRG 336 (transurethral resection of the prostate, patients aged greater than sixty-nine or with complications and comorbidities), which have Medicare cost weights of 0.8929, 1.7771, and 0.9937, respectively. Clearly,

---

1. The relative cost weights are based on the charges hospitals set on the services provided for Medicare patients. In essence, HCFA calculates the average charges (adjusted for location and the indirect costs of graduate medical education) for each DRG. The relative cost for a given DRG is set by dividing the average adjusted charge in a given DRG by the average adjusted charge for all patients across DRGs.

the hospital with a higher percentage of cases in DRG 121 has higher costs than a hospital with a higher percentage in DRG 90.

Assume that hospital A has 1,000 admissions, of which 70 percent are in DRG 90, 10 percent are in DRG 121, and 20 percent are in DRG 336, while hospital B also has 1,000 admissions, of which 20 percent are in DRG 90, 60 percent are in DRG 121, and 20 percent are in DRG 336. If both hospitals are located in the same geographic area (i.e., have the same standardized costs) and if both have the same size teaching programs, then hospital A's revenues from Medicare would be 44 percent higher than hospital B's.

The PPS is not a static reimbursement scheme. In fact, its design has been modified several times since its inception. Some changes have been made because better data have become available, while other modifications have been made in response to political pressures. The two most significant changes in structure have been the gradual reduction in the indirect adjustment for graduate medical education (see chapter 4) and the addition of an adjustment for disproportionate share hospitals (see chapter 6)—hospitals that admit relatively more patients on Medicaid.

The prospective payment system represents a fundamental change in the way hospitals are paid for Medicare patients. Unlike the situation under cost-based reimbursement, hospitals are at risk and can earn profits or incur losses on Medicare patients. A hospital's profits or losses are based on how much it is paid in aggregate. Each year, there is considerable discussion regarding the method used to set the overall payment rate. More important, however, is how PPS sets rates for individual patients. The profit or loss for caring for a given patient depends on how similar that patient is to the average patient discharged in a given DRG as well as the extent to which the treatment technology used is similar to that used for calculating the cost of the average patient. Aggregate profits or losses depend on how close the hospital's actual cost per case is to the average PPS payment. This will depend on whether, on average, the patients the hospital discharges from each DRG are similar to the average across hospitals, on how physicians' practice patterns compare to the average, and on how well the adjustment factors account for the nature of the costs actually incurred by the hospitals (see chapter 7). All of this can lead to either patient dumping or the selection of "profitable" patients.

Medicaid

In reimbursing hospitals for care provided to Medicaid recipients, most states originally followed Medicare methods (i.e., retrospective cost-

Table 2-2.   Basic Features of the Medicaid Hospital Payment System, 1985

Program Characteristics	Number of States
Retrospective cost reimbursement	13
Negotiated rates	2
Per diem: rate increase control, no PGC	7
Per diem: rate increase control, with PGC	9
Per case: rate increase control, no PGC	6
Per case: rate increase control, with PGC	1
DRG case mix	7
Percent of charges: with aggregate budget control	4
Not elsewhere classified	2
PGC, no peer group ceilings	

Source: Adapted from Laudicina, 1985.

based reimbursement). Although states could use different rules to pay providers, they had to secure waivers from the Health Care Financing Administration (HCFA) to do so. These waivers were often difficult to obtain. In 1981, the Congress passed the Omnibus Budget Reconciliation Act, which greatly facilitated the states' ability to implement alternative payment systems. In 1980, thirty-nine states reimbursed hospitals on the basis of retrospective cost-based reimbursement; by 1985, only seven states continued to use such an approach (Laudicina, 1985).

Table 2-2 provides summary descriptive information on the Medicaid hospital payment systems in effect in 1985. All states with prospective payment plans set limits on the rate of increase in Medicaid rates. In most states, the allowable rate of increase was based on the rate of increase either in the cost of the hospital's market basket or in the consumer price index. It is difficult to make a broad generalization about Medicaid rates. Since most states used either the hospital's base-year costs or the hospital's grouping, it is unlikely that any particular category was placed at a disadvantage. However, many hospitals and many analysts have argued that Medicaid rates often do not cover the cost of treating Medicaid patients (Etheredge, 1986; Ginsberg and Sloan, 1984).

Private Third-Party Payors

Private third-party payors include Blue Cross plans, commercial insurance companies, and self-insured firms. Self-insured firms frequently contract with private insurance companies for the management of the health plan offered to their employees. Commercial insurance companies and self-insured plans generally pay hospitals charges (or some percentage thereof) for providing services to their covered populations. Blue Cross plans, which often receive a special discount from hospitals, make payments based on hospital charges or on retrospective costs.

Although the majority of third-party payors reimburses hospitals based on charges or costs, a number of them now negotiate rates with hospitals. This increased aggressiveness on the part of third-party payors is a response to the employers' desire to control the costs of providing medical care to their employees. In particular, health maintenance organizations (HMOs) that do not own their own hospitals, other capitated health systems, comprehensive medical plans (CMPs), and preferred provider organizations (PPOs) often negotiate rates with hospitals. These rates are below the hospital's regular charges. In addition, HMOs, CMPs, and PPOs often negotiate with a subset of hospitals in a given community and consequently either direct their subscribers to those hospitals or give them strong financial incentives to use them.

Source of Payment

This brief discussion of methods of paying hospitals indicates that a hospital's net patient revenues depends on the type of health insurance coverage its patients have as well as the state in which it is located. In general, the ratio of net revenues to actual patient charges will be highest for patients covered by commercial health insurance companies, next highest for patients covered by Blue Cross Plans, and lowest for people covered by Medicaid. Given the structure of the Medicare prospective payment system, Medicare payments may exceed charges in some hospitals but be lower than them in other hospitals.

Table 2-3 presents data on the source of patient revenue by the four categories of hospitals. These data are based on information on the expected primary source of payment recorded by the hospital when the patient was admitted. Compared to other hospitals, major COTH hospitals admit more patients who are self-paying or from whom the hospital expects to receive either no payment or reduced payment. Many patients in the first group may leave the hospital with

Table 2-3.   Sources of Patient Revenue, by Type of Hospital, 1981 (percent)

Payment Source	Major COTH				Minor COTH			
	All	Public	Not for Profit	For Profit	All	Public	Not for Profit	For Profit
Self-pay	11.68	17.18	6.36	32.47	6.71	20.31	6.03	4.82
Medicare	19.81	15.83	23.35	17.02	26.97	15.72	27.59	24.43
Medicaid	16.79	20.66	13.49	14.08	12.04	23.89	11.53	5.73
Blue Cross	18.98	10.59	26.48	11.22	27.47	14.07	28.17	27.35
Commercial insurance	19.12	15.15	22.67	15.46	20.99	10.95	21.31	33.84
Reduced or no charge	17.79	28.94	7.65	34.50	8.30	26.40	7.40	5.31

Source: Based on data from American Hospital Association, A, 1985; U.S. Department of Health & Human Services, 1981a.

bad debts; the latter patients are identified in advance as being probable charity patients.

When hospitals are further disaggregated by ownership, a different picture emerges. Relative to all other hospitals, more patients at public teaching hospitals (both COTH and non-COTH) are without insurance and more are eligible for Medicaid. With respect to expected source of payment for patients, not-for-profit COTH hospitals are more similar to nonteaching hospitals than they are to public COTH hospitals.

Changes in Source of Payment

Table 2-4 provides data on the source of revenue for 1980 and 1984 for three groups of hospitals. Unfortunately, we were unable to disaggregate COTH hospitals either into major and minor categories or into level of control. The bases for the distributions in tables 2-3 and 2-4 are different. Table 2-3 presents data on the distribution of *patients* within each group of hospitals, while table 2-4 presents data on the distribution of *revenue*. For example, since the average Medicare patient stays longer than the average patient and has more costly illnesses, Medicare revenues represent a higher proportion of total revenues than Medicare patients do of total patients.

In terms of revenue distribution, the major difference across the three groups of hospitals is that Medicaid represents a higher proportion of patient revenue in COTH hospitals than in the other hospitals. This is consistent with the data on the distribution of patients shown in table 2-3. The data in table 2-4 suggest that there was a significant

Other Teaching				Nonteaching			
All	Public	Not for Profit	For Profit	All	Public	Not for Profit	For Profit
6.51	11.13	5.81	4.31	6.48	8.35	6.00	5.52
26.78	20.51	27.44	34.00	31.81	34.18	30.67	32.78
9.41	14.28	8.81	5.10	8.69	9.64	8.33	8.65
21.00	12.70	22.42	22.84	19.09	14.91	21.78	14.64
28.36	23.93	29.10	29.44	28.75	27.78	27.99	33.31
8.93	24.20	6.38	4.70	7.17	9.32	6.66	5.92

shift in the source of revenue between 1980 and 1984 for all groups of hospitals. On a relative basis, revenues from self-paying and Medicare patients increased, while revenues from Medicaid and private insurance fell. Many factors can account for this switch—including the decrease in admissions in the population under age sixty-five, increases in the proportion of the population without health insurance, and a tightening of Medicaid payment rates—all of which occurred during that time period.

Financial Arrangements between Teaching Hospitals and Related Institutions

Although the data presented in table 2-1 indicate that only 10 percent of the revenues of COTH hospitals come from nonpatient sources, this may be an underestimate of the support that teaching hospitals receive to support functions other than patient care. Some of the resources used to support services provided in teaching hospitals are not recorded on the financial statements of hospitals. There are two basic reasons for this:

1. COTH hospitals are often part of academic medical centers, and the flow of resources between the institutions that make up that center are complicated and governed by complex bargaining procedures.
2. Some of the teaching and research is done by physicians and scientists who are not paid by the hospital or any other organization for performing that function. Rather, they provide these services in return for benefits, either psychological or economic.

Table 2-4.   Sources of Patient Revenue, by Type of Hospital, 1980 and 1984

Payment Source	COTH		Other Teaching		Nonteaching	
	1980	1984	1980	1984	1980	1984
Private insurance	46.4	43.6	48.0	44.8	46.9	43.8
Medicare	32.4	39.6	35.5	40.3	37.0	40.8
Medicaid	13.6	10.6	11.3	6.9	7.3	7.1
Patient	7.5	8.1	5.3	8.0	8.8	8.3

Source: Based on data from Georgetown University Center for Health Policy.

Neither the cost of the services provided or the benefits received are recorded as financial flows between hospitals and physicians.

These two issues are discussed in more detail below.

Understanding the financial arrangements that take place within the academic health center is important when considering how individual services are financed. A review of some of these arrangements demonstrates both the complexity and some of the difficulties created by current methods of financing.

Figure 2-1 shows the various interactions that may occur between the teaching hospital and other entities, both within and outside of the academic medical center. Within the academic medical center, teaching hospitals interact with various components of the university, with physicians, and with clinics. Outside the academic medical center, the teaching hospital may interact with other teaching hospitals, including Veterans Administration hospitals and a multitude of federal and state agencies. This figure was drawn several years ago; the growth since then of HMOs, PPOs, and multi-institutional systems adds a further dimension of complexity to the flow of funds between teaching hospitals and related internal and external organizations.

Arthur Young (1987) used figure 2-1 as a guide to studying the financial arrangements of thirty-six teaching hospitals during 1983 and 1984. The flow of revenues was to determine the magnitude of the flow of funds into and out of teaching hospitals. Also, numerous hospital administrators were interviewed concerning negotiated or noncash transactions. Results from this study suggest that the financial arrangements are unique to each teaching hospital and that few general statements can be made about flow of funds.

The Arthur Young study found that many physicians served without pay as faculty members in graduate medical education programs and that the implicit costs associated with this service were not re-

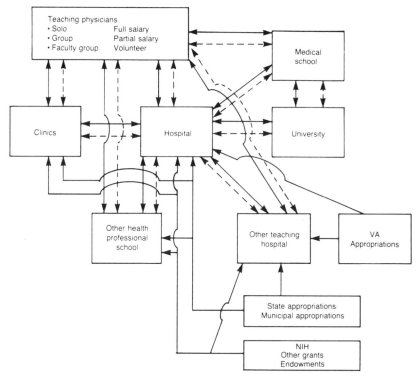

Figure 2-1.   A Schematic of the Flow of Hospital Costs, Revenues, and Services
    Source: Arthur Young, 1986a.

corded on any financial statement. In thirty-three of thirty-six teaching hospitals studied by Arthur Young, physicians donated some portion of their time for the instruction of residents. Donated time is defined as time for which the physician neither was paid by the hospital nor earned a professional fee. In more than half of teaching hospitals, faculty donated more than 20 percent of their time for the education of residents. The study also found that the percentage of donated time increased as the number of residents in the hospital declined. This suggests that hospitals with one or two residency programs rely primarily on part-time, community physicians for residency education.

The value of a physician's donated time is considerable. In one hospital, eighty attending physicians donated an average of 250 hours per physician per year for residency education. Assuming average hourly earnings of $50, this represents a physician contribution of $1 million to the educational program of that hospital. In another hospital, the physician contribution was estimated to be $1.3 million.

The Arthur Young study documented that a portion of graduate medical education costs is paid indirectly by attending physicians, who use faculty practice plan revenues to support clinical education. Approximately half of the faculty practice plans studied by Arthur Young had a fund that was used for equipment purchases, fellowship programs, house officers' travel to conferences, and other educational activities. The extent of support by faculty practice plans varied substantially by hospital and by its residency program.

The cost of graduate medical education borne by physicians rather than by hospitals is evidently quite considerable. Arthur Young, however, made no effort to document the benefits physicians received for being on a graduate medical faculty. Potential benefits are increased professional productivity and increased income, especially if their enhanced prestige from association with a teaching hospital enables them to raise their fees. Further, their involvement with young inquiring minds carries its own benefit.

Arthur Young found that support for other educational programs by physicians or other health professionals was much more limited. Very little time for the training of nursing or allied health profession students was donated by hospital personnel. In addition, teaching hospitals rarely received outside financial assistance for the training of medical, nursing, or allied health professions students. Many of these students performed services that may have covered all of the cost of their training.

The arrangements to finance research projects is perhaps even more complex than those that finance clinical education. In most academic medical centers, the medical school receives a grant from the National Institutes of Health, a pharmaceutical company, or other source. The grant theoretically covers the full direct cost of conducting the research and allows for overhead costs. The allowance for overhead can be as much as 40 percent of the direct cost of the project. As discussed in chapter 5, it is unclear whether the hospital receives its full share of the direct cost, since the incremental costs of research protocols on patient care services are frequently unknown. In some academic medical centers, the hospital receives a share of the overhead from the grant, while in others the medical school retains all of the overhead. Some teaching hospitals have established separate entities to sponsor research projects and thereby receive all the reimbursement for overhead expenses.

Support for other functions in the teaching hospital are much more idiosyncratic, and thus it is more difficult to generalize about support for these functions. Most university-owned hospitals receive an allocation of the university's endowment income. These are discretionary funds that may be used to support individual research projects or to cover an operating deficit.

Hospitals generally provide funds to other entities in the academic medical center on a contractual basis. For example, the chair of the department of radiology in the medical school may also be the head of the radiology department in the hospital. In most institutions, the medical school or faculty practice plan pays the salary of faculty members and is reimbursed by the hospital for time spent managing the hospital department. In examining these relationships, Arthur Young concluded that in most cases the contractual arrangements were negotiated at cost to each entity.

The flow of funds between teaching hospitals and other hospitals, such as Veterans Administration or community hospitals, is unique to each arrangement. The general perception is that hospitals with large teaching programs allow their residents to rotate to hospitals with smaller educational programs without charging those hospitals for a portion of their salaries. This was found in most but not all hospitals in the Arthur Young study. However, this practice may be changing as number of residents becomes an increasingly important factor in Medicare payments. Another general perception is that Veterans Administration hospitals support the teaching hospitals with which they are affiliated. This was not substantiated by the Arthur Young study, although the number of affiliated relationships studied was relatively small.

Hospital Financial Viability

As indicated above, there have been major changes in the 1980s in the rules governing third-party payments to hospitals. The most significant change is the shift under Medicare and some Medicaid programs from retrospective cost-based reimbursement to prospective payment. This means that hospitals can now incur substantial profits or losses for taking care of these patients. At the same time, the private sector is taking action to encourage price competition among hospitals and to limit its obligations for hospital services.

In spite of, or perhaps because of, the turmoil in the hospital environment, overall hospital margins increased from 1980 to 1986, and operating margins at teaching hospitals exceeded those of non-teaching hospitals (American Hospital Association, 1987b). In fact, in most of these years the operating margins of teaching hospitals exceeded those of nonteaching hospitals by one or two percentage points. The better financial performance of teaching hospitals can be attributed to several factors, of which two are most important: the profits they earned under Medicare PPS and their ability to increase their market share in a declining market. In this chapter, we discuss the increase in profits experienced during the first two years of PPS. In chapter 3, we examine the change in market shares across the four groups of hospitals.

The Effect of PPS

One major source of overall hospital profits between 1984 and 1986 was the profits the hospitals earned for providing services to Medicare patients. During congressional hearings in February 1987, three representatives from government agencies stated that hospitals were earning profits on Medicare patients of between 12 and 16 percent during 1984 and 1985. Each reported that teaching hospitals had higher operating margins than nonteaching hospitals. For example, the Prospective Payment Assessment Commission found that 1984 profit margins under PPS were 21.1 percent for major teaching hospitals, 16.7 percent for other teaching hospitals, and 12.4 percent for nonteaching hospitals (Altman, 1987). However, those margins fell considerably in the third year of PPS (ProPAC, 1988a).

The high Medicare profits in the first years of PPS, which were somewhat unexpected, are attributable to a number of interrelated factors (Gordon, 1988). The initial rates, which were based on unaudited data, may have been set above their target—the estimated average cost per case in 1984. At the same time, hospitals responded to the new payment system by decreasing lengths of stay, shifting certain services to an outpatient basis, coding cases more accurately, and changing hospital service patterns (Gutterman and Dobson, 1986). The higher profits realized by teaching hospitals are partly due to the fact that the initial adjustment for the indirect costs of graduate medical education, which increased DRG payments by over 11 percent for each 0.1 percent increase in the residents per bed ratio, overcompensated hospitals for these costs (Lave, 1985). This adjustment was higher than any estimate of the indirect costs determined by estimated hospital cost functions.[2]

The Future

The recent past may not be a good guide to what will happen to hospitals' financial status in the future. The healthy financial conditions of 1984 and 1985 have begun to deteriorate. Many of the factors that led to high Medicare profits and thus to overall hospital profitability have been eliminated. Easy adjustments in hospitals' practice patterns have been made as have changes in coding practices. The increase in the overall PPS rate has been held below the increase in the prices that hospitals have to pay for their inputs—the hospital market basket—for four years. The adjustment for indirect costs of graduate medical education have been reduced, eliminating a source of excess profits for hospitals with large teaching programs. Experts argue that without a change in policy, Medicare margins will approach zero in 1988 (Altman, 1987; Dobson and Hoy, 1988).

The outlook for hospitals does not look any more optimistic if we examine the policies likely to be pursued by other payors. Medicaid programs, which already pay low rates, are likely to continue to be very restrictive in their payments. Other third-party payors will continue to look for mechanisms to contain their expenditures. These mechanisms are discussed in more detail in the chapters to follow. In chapters 7 through 10, we propose some changes in policy to remedy the shortcomings of current policies.

---

2. Some of the excess profits may be due to the fact that the hospital-specific component of the standardized rate was set too high. The problem arose from the fact that the estimated hospital case mix index, which was based on reported 1981 diagnostic data, may have been too low. (For example, some major teaching hospitals did not report secondary diagnoses.) The hospital-specific component was determined by dividing the hospital's costs by its DRG index. If the index was "too low," its standardized costs would be "too high."

part II | Policy Issues

In chapters 3–6 we discuss four hospital services: patient care (chapter 3), clinical education (chapter 4), biomedical research (chapter 5), and care of uninsured patients (chapter 6). We begin each chapter with a historical perspective. It is our belief that many policy debates have been constrained by the evolution of the delivery system and that, in order to fully understand the available options, a historical perspective is necessary. With this background, we then examine issues of cost, financing, distribution, and control.

Although it is frequently difficult to obtain a precise estimate of the cost of each service because many of the services are produced jointly, there have been numerous attempts to estimate the cost of individual services. For each service, we review the available studies and attempt to derive a consensus estimate of the cost of each service. For certain services, it is necessary to analyze new data in order to obtain estimates.

The methods of financing the various services are extremely complex. Hospitals, third-party payors, and governments have developed elaborate systems to support each service. Each of these services is cross-subsidized heavily. We will attempt to identify how each service is funded. None of the services is distributed equally across all hospitals. Each service is highly concentrated in a relatively few hospitals, although it is unclear how much overlap there is among hospitals in the provision of each service.

Who controls the provision of services is a major concern for hospital administrators and policy makers. In the past, most of the control has rested with administrators and professional societies, and most of the payments have come from third parties. As payment reforms become more stringent, the locus of control may shift to the payors.

chapter 3 | Patient Care

The twentieth century has been a period of dramatic and dynamic change for the hospital sector. At the beginning of the century, hospitals were primarily infirmaries where the poor received shelter. With improved education of physicians and hospital personnel and numerous scientific advances, hospitals developed into modern scientific institutions where people from all walks of life went to receive care. During the twentieth century, major initiatives to improve access to hospitals and upgrade facilities were launched.

After years of expansion, the hospital industry is now beset by a different set of conditions. A result of increase in capacity is that competition among hospitals for patients has increased. In addition, alternative providers, such as free-standing surgical and diagnostic centers, are now treating the kinds of patients who once were the hospitals' sole responsibility. Added to this competition are the aggressive actions being taken by the payors of hospital services, both public and private, to try to control their expenditures for hospital services.

In this chapter, we discuss the growth of the hospital sector and especially the factors promoting the expansion of patient care services. We examine the capacity of the nation's hospitals for producing patient care services and the distribution of patients across the different categories of hospitals. Next, we discuss the costs of providing patient care services and the accompanying sources of patient care revenue. We then go on to examine a number of control mechanisms that payors and hospitals have implemented to influence patient access to hospital services and the types of services provided to certain patients. Finally, we return to an issue discussed briefly in chapter 2, that is, the effect that the changes during the 1980s have had on the distribution of patients among types of hospitals.

Background

When hospitals were first established in the United States in the eighteenth century, they were designed to provide services for people who could not obtain medical care elsewhere. They were predominantly almshouses, which offered treatment to the insane, patients without families, and other individuals who could not be treated at home. Most Americans received their medical care in their homes; hospitals were considered dangerous places.

Since the mid-nineteenth century, the American hospital sector has experienced significant transformation and growth (Starr, 1982). The transformation can best be described by labels used to characterize the hospital. The hospital, once known as a house of despair became a house of hope. It evolved from a custodial institution into a complex scientific institution at the heart of the health care industry (Knowles, 1977).

This evolution of the hospital sector was stimulated by the growing awareness that hospital inpatient services could make a significant difference in health outcomes. Improvements in anesthesiology and the development of methods to control infections made hospitals the preferred location for surgery. As quality of care improved, the affluent began to shift their locus of care from the home to the hospital. Illness, rather than social class, became the motivating reason for admission to the hospital. Other changes, such as increases in income, urbanization, and changing family structure brought health care services into the hospital. Services that were once provided in the home by family members were now being purchased from physicians, hospitals, and other health care providers. By the early twentieth century, hospitals had become the institutions of choice for medical treatment.

As the twentieth century progressed, several initiatives were designed to promote access to hospital services. At the beginning of the century, the federal government and many state governments introduced workman's compensation programs to cover the medical expenses of injured workers. Private insurance to protect individuals against the cost of hospital care, first introduced in 1929, spread rapidly during World War II, when it became a nontaxable employee fringe benefit. Employer-based health insurance, which became a standard part of employee benefit packages, made coverage available to millions of employees and their dependents.

In response to the growing demand for hospital services, the federal government initiated a number of programs designed to increase access to the hospital. For example, the implementation of the Hospital Survey and Construction Act of 1946 (the Hill-Burton program), which spent $3.7 billion for the construction and modernization of hospitals between 1947 and 1972, was partially responsible for the rapid growth in the number of hospital beds that took place in the 1950s (Lave and Lave, 1974).

Expansion of the capacity and capability of the hospital system was followed by public policies to increase access to the system by the poor and the elderly. In the 1950s, the federal government began to share in the cost of direct payments to providers—referred to as vendor payments—for services provided to recipients of federal categorical assistance programs (Lave, 1967). In 1960, the Kerr-Mills program expanded the vendor payment programs for low-income elderly. Finally, in 1965 the Medicare and Medicaid programs, which superseded the earlier, more limited programs, made health coverage available to millions of low-income and elderly persons (Somers and Somers, 1967).

The structure of both private and public health insurance programs further stimulated the growth of the hospital sector (Feldstein, 1971; Feldstein, 1977; Newhouse, 1978). The hospitalized patient was likely to have fairly complete coverage for both hospital and physician services. For example, by 1970 approximately 89 percent of expenditures for hospital services were paid for through third parties (Waldo, Lewit, and Lazenby, 1986). As a result, most patients were unaffected by the cost of care provided in hospitals and had few incentives to seek low-cost providers. In addition, the methods third parties used to reimburse hospitals were generally considered to be inflationary. Hospitals were reimbursed either on the basis of submitted charges or incurred costs, determined retrospectively. In essence, the hospitals were given a blank check to set their own prices and determine their costs, while the individual patient was relatively unaffected by the cost.

The expansion of the hospital sector is underscored by the fact that, between 1967 and 1985, the annual rate of growth of expenditures on hospital services was 18.4 percent. Although some of that growth is accounted for by a growing and aging population and by general inflation in the economy, almost one-third of the increase is due to changes in the nature of the hospital product. Service intensity (the change in the nature of the hospital product) is a generic term that covers the use of more personnel and ancillary services as well as the use of new diagnostic and treatment technologies to treat new and existing medical problems. Several studies indicate that, between 1967 and 1985, service intensity increased by about four percentage points per year and accounted for about one-third of the increase in expenditures on hospital care (Anderson, 1986; U.S. Congress, Office of Technology Assessment, 1984).

The growth of the hospital system was accompanied by an increase in health care expenditures by public agencies and private organizations. Between 1973 and 1982, expenditures for hospital services under the Medicare program increased at an annual rate of 17 percent, while expenditures for hospital services by Medicaid programs increased at an annual rate of 14.1 percent. At the same time, the cost of providing health insurance for employees and their dependents became a major business expense for employers. During the 1980s, both public and private sectors began to search for mechanisms to control their health care expenditures and to turn open-ended obligations into controllable expenses.

The efforts of payors to control their expenditures for hospital services received support from researchers investigating various aspects of the health care delivery system. First, research findings suggested that a considerable amount of care provided in hospitals was inappropriate—that either the admission itself was not appropriate (the patient could have been cared for in different settings), the length of stay was unnecessarily long, or unnecessary services were provided (Gertman and Restuccia, 1981; Payne, 1987). Second, studies indicated that there were no incentives for hospitals to be managed efficiently and that there was a considerable amount of waste in the system (Newhouse, 1978). Indeed, under cost-based reimbursement, a hospital that tried to control costs was rewarded with a reduction in revenue. Third, some researchers argued that the contribution to health status resulting from increased service intensity may not have been worth the cost (Fuchs, 1974). Most of these negative findings were attributed in large part to the structure of health insurance and the mechanisms for paying providers. Finally, alternative forms of delivering health care, such as health maintenance organizations, were cheaper and just as effective. One implication of the research results was that it should be possible to decrease the costs of hospital care without significantly decreasing access to the hospital system or the quality of care provided.

The initial efforts to control expenditures for hospital services— certificate-of-need programs, comprehensive health planning, and development of formal utilization review programs—were undertaken soon after rising hospital costs became a major public policy issue. Evaluations of these approaches indicated that they were not very effective (Salkever and Bice, 1976). Consequently, strong pressures ensued to search for policies that would lead to more fundamental changes in the way health care services were produced and delivered. These policies can be classified into four different types of initiatives.

The first set of policies were directed at changing the way providers, particularly hospitals, are paid for rendering services. A variety of prospective payment systems were designed to increase the efficiency with which hospitals are managed and to control the overall growth of the hospital sector. The second set of policies was designed to increase enrollment in capitated health care systems, such as HMOs. The third set of policies changed the amount of cost sharing that individuals faced in their insurance policies. Finally, a set of policies—represented by the development of second-opinion surgery programs, preadmission screening, case-management, and so on—was designed to control unnecessary hospital utilization.

While these various policies were being implemented, the number of alternative providers—organizations now rendering services that once could be provided only in a hospital—also increased. These alternative providers include surgical centers, alternative birthing centers, and diagnostic centers. This expansion in alternative providers was partially due to the tremendous increase in health care personnel (nurses, psychologists, physicians, etc.) who were trained in the 1970s in programs funded by the federal government. Alternative providers compete directly with hospitals for patients.

All of these factors—government sponsorship of increased capacity of the health care sector followed by hospital payment reform, increasing management of health care utilization, and increased competition—have left the hospital sector with excess capacity. The outward indicator of excess capacity is the low and falling average hospital occupancy rate. As shown in table 3-1, the overall hospital occupancy rate has fallen from 75.4 percent in 1980 to 64.3 in 1986. The drop in occupancy has occurred because, while admission and inpatient days per 1,000 population have fallen continuously since 1980, the number of beds per capita has changed very little (Anderson, 1988).

Excess capacity is both a cause and a consequence of the reforms that have taken place. Without the slack in capacity, it is unlikely that governments and businesses would have been able to implement cost containment policies. If hospitals faced an excess demand for their services, they would have no need to negotiate prices, to participate

Table 3-1. Indicators of Excess Hospital Capacity, Short-Term Community Hospitals, 1980–1986

Year	Hospital Occupancy Rates	Hospital Beds per Capita (1,000 pop.)	Hospital Admissions per Thousand	Hospital Days per Thousand
1980	75.4	3.918	153.8	1,169.17
1981	75.9	4.234	153.5	1,166.33
1982	75.2	4.225	151.9	1,152.62
1983	73.4	4.210	149.3	1,134.55
1984	68.9	4.168	143.9	1,050.16
1985	64.8	4.191	140.1	991.18
1986	64.3	4.056	134.3	951.69

Source: Based on data from American Hospital Association, 1987a, table 6.

in preferred provider arrangements, or to enter into contracts with HMOs. The implementation of a Medicare prospective payment system would have been difficult to achieve if the major policy concern was whether or not hospitals would admit Medicare patients.

The situation that hospitals find themselves in is therefore very different from that which existed in the 1970s. Excess capacity has replaced shortages. Constrained financing systems have replaced open-ended systems. These changes will influence the kinds of services that hospitals provide and how they provide them, and it is worth stressing that many of these policies were implemented in order to change the way that services were provided in hospitals.

With this background, we now turn to various dimensions of patient care in the second half of the 1980s.

Distribution

In 1986, there were nearly 32 million admissions to community hospitals. As indicated in table 3-2, 8 percent of these admissions were to major COTH hospitals, 13 percent to minor COTH hospitals, 29 percent to other teaching hospitals, and 50 percent to nonteaching hospitals. As we discuss below, the types of patients treated in each of these categories of hospitals differ, with major and minor COTH hospitals being more likely to admit patients with conditions needing longer lengths of stay. This explains the different patterns of inpatient days. The data on distribution of beds indicate that beds are used

Table 3-2.   Distribution of Patient Activity, by Type of Hospital, 1986 (percent)

Utilization	Major COTH	Minor COTH	Other Teaching	Nonteaching
Admissions	8.04	13.20	29.00	49.76
Inpatient days	9.41	14.31	28.64	47.54
Emergency Room visits	7.69	11.77	27.28	53.26
All Outpatient visits	11.42	16.21	27.56	44.81
Beds	7.75	12.24	26.95	52.96

Source: Based on data from American Hospital Association, A, 1986.

more intensively in teaching hospitals than in nonteaching hospitals, and thus that their occupancy rates are higher.

In 1986 short-term general hospitals reported 225 million out-patient visits and 75 million visits to emergency rooms. The distribution of emergency room visits across the four groups of hospitals is very similar to that of admissions and inpatient days. However, the distribution of outpatient visits is somewhat different. Relative to admissions, both major and minor COTH hospitals reported more out-patient visits.

Patient Characteristics

There is considerable variation across hospitals regarding the scope of services that they offer. Table 3-3 shows various services by hospital category. On average, major COTH hospitals offered thirty-nine of the fifty-nine services covered in the survey, minor COTH hospitals offered thirty-six, other teaching hospitals offered twenty-six, and nonteaching hospitals offered only fifteen. The availability of specific facilities and services shows even greater variation. Burn care units, neonatal intensive care units, open-heart surgery, and transplant capacity are all much more likely to be found in major COTH hospitals.

Given the differences in the number and kinds of services available, we would expect the types of patients treated to vary across the four groups of hospitals. While the existence of a service does not necessarily mean that the service is used intensively or even appropriately, the lack of a service precludes a hospital from admitting certain patients. Obviously, open-heart surgery can be done only in hospitals that have heart-lung machines. In addition to being equipped to treat patients with conditions that cannot be treated elsewhere, the major teaching hospitals are staffed by academic physicians, whose

Table 3-3.   Facilities and Services, by Type of Hospital (percent)

Hospital Facility or Service	Major COTH	Minor COTH	Other Teaching	Nonteaching	All Hospitals
AIDS services	91	80	55	20	29
Cardiac catheter lab	94	85	45	8	19
CT scanner	98	95	82	49	57
Diagnostic radioisotope facility	96	95	87	54	61
Extracorporeal lithotripter	25	12	5	1	3
Fertility counseling	75	55	17	3	8
Genetic counseling	77	50	12	1	6
Hemodialysis	91	87	55	16	26
Radioactive implant facility	89	82	49	13	23
Megavoltage radiation facility	84	74	37	7	16
NMR imaging facility	52	24	11	3	6
Open-heart surgery capability	89	63	30	3	12
Organ transplant capability	75	23	8	1	4
Therapeutic radioisotope	91	84	50	12	23
Trauma center	78	60	36	12	19
X-ray radiation therapy	82	73	38	8	17

Source: Based on data from American Hospital Association, A, 1986.

clinical knowledge is at the frontier of medicine (Lewis and Sheps, 1983; Rogers, 1978). Thus, these hospitals often serve as major referral institutions, drawing their patient population from beyond the boundaries of the counties or states in which they are located.

While the patients admitted to these four categories of hospitals differ, the important question is, How different? Here, we explore five approaches to determining this.

Diagnosis-Related Groups

Thousands of diseases and conditions may necessitate hospitalization. Patients may have mild or severe manifestations of a problem; they may have comorbid conditions that exacerbate the precipitating problem or may suffer complications while in the hospital. Patients may be treated medically or surgically. They may enter the hospital with a diagnosis well established, or it may be necessary to establish the diagnosis during hospitalization. To compare the types of patients treated in different hospitals, some way of describing the patient population succinctly is necessary (Hornbrook, 1982).

At present, the most frequently used summary statistic describing a hospital's inpatient population is the DRG-based case mix index (Fetter, 1982; Pettingill and Vertrees, 1982). To create this index, the proportion of a hospital's inpatient population that falls into each DRG is determined. The DRG proportion is then multiplied by the (estimated) relative cost of treating patients in each DRG (see chapter 1 and below) and the weighted proportions are then summed. The resulting index is a measure of the relative costliness of a hospital's inpatient population.

Other Aggregate Patient Mix Measures

The DRGs, which provide the basis for the DRG-based case mix index, have been strongly criticized as a patient classification system. One argument is that they do not account for patient complexity and that, consequently, they may underestimate the differences in the types of patients seen in different types of hospitals. In particular, many hypothesize that teaching hospitals are more likely to admit complex patients. Before looking at current data relating to this hypothesis, it is worthwhile to spend a little more time reviewing the criticisms of DRGs.

Critics argue that DRGs are not clinically homogeneous; that is, DRGs group together patients who are dissimilar with respect to their clinical status and thus their treatment needs (Horn et al., 1986). Although the debate over heterogeneity within the DRGs is quite complex, there are essentially two aspects of the debate. Some critics believe that DRG groupings are fundamentally flawed; that is, they combine people in the same patient group who should in fact be in separate categories. Others believe that DRG groups are incomplete; that is, they group patients who vary with respect to the severity of their condition and this variation should be taken into consideration. They argue that the DRGs should be disaggregated further. For example, patients within a given DRG who have organ failure should be in a different subgroup than patients classified into that DRG but without organ failure.

Four other patient classification systems have received considerable attention as either supplements for or complements to the DRG patient classification system. These are the severity of illness index (Horn, Horn, and Sharkey, 1984); patient management categories (Young et al., 1983); disease staging (Gonnella, Hornbrook, and Lewis, 1984); and MEDISGRP (Brewster et al., 1985). Two of these systems (severity of illness and MEDISGRPS) use physiological and test information reported in the patient's medical record to assign a patient a score, which is an indicator of the patient's acuity or severity level. The severity of illness index is diagnosis specific, whereas the MEDISGRPS index is not.

Patient management categories (PMCs), like DRGs, group patients together depending on the diagnoses and procedures listed on the discharge abstract. However, the approach taken to construct PMCs was quite different than that taken to construct DRGs. The developers of PMCs worked with physicians first to develop groups of patients who were expected to need similar hospital services. Then the researchers examined the *International Classification of Diseases— Ninth Revision* (ICD-9) to assign codes to the patients clustered in each group. The developers of DRGs, on the other hand, worked with physicians to assign all ICD-9 diagnoses into major diagnostic categories, to subdivide these further into medical and surgical cases, and to subdivide them even further into additional categories.

Disease staging measures the severity of the patient's condition at a given point in time according to five clinically identifiable stages in the progression of the disease. Staging uses information either from the patient's medical record or from the discharge abstract.

Few reports in the literature indicate the difference each of these grouping systems make in describing patients. A study of patients in New York found that severity of illness was higher in teaching hospitals than in nonteaching hospitals (Berman et al., 1986). Analyses of the distribution of patients classified by the disease-staging methods in both New York (Berman et al., 1986) and Maryland hospitals (Coffey and Goldfarb, 1986) did not find that stage of illness varied significantly with extent of teaching. Horn et al. (1985) found that, although teaching hospitals frequently treat a higher proportion of severely ill patients, the distribution of severity levels among study hospitals was not predicted reliably by hospital type or by the ratio of interns and residents to beds. Finally, the Arthur Young study (1986b) found that the overall severity of illness did not vary systematically across categories of hospitals.

In summary, analyses to date do not indicate that the average level of patient severity varies across the four types of hospitals. This result does not settle any of the issues raised above with respect to the strengths or weaknesses of any of the classification systems.

Case-Mix Commonality

The third measure of case mix variation is commonality—the extent to which the mix of patients differs from one hospital to another. While

Table 3-4.   Patients by Type of Hospital and Diagnosis-Related Group in California

Characteristic	Major COTH	Minor COTH	Other Teaching	Nonteaching
Overall Case Mix Index	1.15	1.10	1.02	.94
Twenty most common DRGs	32.6	38.6	39.4	36.4
Fifty most common DRGs	1.5	0.9	.7	.7
Patients receiving hospital care in county of residence	70.2	77.7	78.9	79.3

Source: Based on data from California Health Facilities, 1983.

the case mix index provides information on whether one hospital's case mix is more expensive, it does not provide any information on the extent to which the patients admitted to different types of hospitals are similar or different. This dimension of case mix is likely to become more important as the hospital industry becomes more competitive. For example, competition among hospitals is likely to be more intense if they admit patients with the same medical conditions.

No published studies report on the proportion of discharges that are common or rare to a category of hospital. However, we were able to calculate such a measure for California hospitals. In order to determine the extent to which groups of hospitals admitted similar or different patients, we calculated the proportion of discharges from California hospitals in 1983 that were assigned to the twenty most common and the fifty least common DRGs for each group of hospitals. As shown in Table 3-4, the most common DRGs made up a smaller percentage of discharges for major COTH hospitals than for the other groups, but the difference was not statistically significant. The fifty least common DRGs constituted a higher proportion of the discharges at teaching hospitals than at nonteaching hospitals. These data indicate that there was considerable overlap in the types of patients treated in all groups of hospitals, although, as expected, the very rare cases are more likely to be treated in the teaching hospitals.

Patient Referrals and Transfers

Patients who are referred to or transferred to a particular institution because of the hospital's reputed expertise may be different from the average patient in a DRG. Referred patients may need a different set of services than the average patient (in the DRG), or they may be referred because they or their physician prefer the type of care provided in the institution to which they were referred. Referrals are generally made by physicians before a patient is admitted to a hospital, and therefore documentation as to how a patient got to a particular hospital is difficult to obtain. Transfers occur for a variety of reasons. One measure of the extent to which a hospital is a referral hospital may be the proportion of the inpatient population that comes from outside of the county in which the hospital is located. Table 3-4 presents such information for hospitals in California. The groups differ with respect to the proportion of patients from outside the county. Major COTH hospitals in California admit a higher proportion of their patients from outside the county than do the other groups of hospitals.

Researchers at the Health Care Financing Administration have also constructed indicators of the extent to which hospitals are referral institutions (Jencks and Bobula, in press). In studying the Medicare inpatient population, HCFA analysts developed a measure indicating whether a patient was a transfer patient (i.e., a patient who was transferred from one hospital to another) or a possible referral patient (a patient admitted to a hospital other than one other persons in his or her place of residence were admitted to). They then determined an index for each hospital, which measures the proportion of patients transferred or referred. Both the transfer index and the referral index were found to be positively correlated with the extent of teaching at a hospital.

Social Case Mix

Both the location and the mission of the hospital influence the types of patient admitted. Because hospitals admit a significant proportion of their patients from their surrounding communities, the socioeconomic characteristics among their patients will differ. Hospitals located in the affluent suburbs will have a different patient population than hospitals located in the inner city. In addition, a hospital's primary mission can be to render services to specific groups; for example, Cook County Hospital's charter is to serve the poor in Chicago.

It is generally believed that the disadvantaged are likely to be sicker when they come into the hospital, because they put off seeing a physician until their illnesses become incapacitating. In addition, such patients may be more difficult to discharge: their home environments may be less conducive to recuperation, and in many cases there may be no one able to provide follow-up care. Some inferences about social case mix can be drawn from the data on primary source of payment presented in table 2-3. Compared to other groups of hospitals, COTH hospitals are more likely to admit Medicaid patients and the uninsured. However, as pointed out in chapter 2, when hospitals are further disaggregated by type of control, it is the public COTH hospitals that admit the disproportionate number of Medicaid and uninsured patients.

Outpatient Population

As indicated by the data in table 3-2, all hospitals engage in significant outpatient activity, with major COTH hospitals providing a large share. Unfortunately, we have no information on the nature of outpatient and emergency room visits, so we have only anecdotal information on how patients in these settings vary across categories of hospitals. Research in the classification of outpatient visits is still in preliminary stages, and no measure comparable to the DRG case mix index exists for ambulatory care. Research in classifying emergency room patients, particularly along dimensions of urgency, is well developed, but to our knowledge there have been no reports on the characteristics of patients by hospital category.

Costs of Patient Care

In 1986 the average cost of a hospital discharge was $3,022 (see table I-1). The average cost varied significantly across hospital groups, from $5,432 at major COTH hospitals to $4,557 at minor COTH hospitals. As discussed in chapter 1, there are many reasons for this difference: the hospitals are located in different labor markets, the hospitals admit and treat different types of patients, or the hospitals' treatment protocols vary. Here, we focus the discussion on two factors that generate differences in the cost—difference in case mix and differences in practice patterns.

Differences in Case Mix

It is well known that the costs of treating different types of patients vary. For example, it is more costly to treat a patient with an acute myocardial infarction (AMI) than it is to treat a simple pneumonia case. Determining precisely how much more it costs to treat the AMI patient is more complicated than it initially appears. There are many different approaches to assessing how costly it is to treat individual patients including

1. Measuring the physical resources used to treat each patient.
2. Using patient charge information, with the assumption that charges reflect costs (Lave and Leinhardt, 1976).
3. Using patient charge information and adjusting it by department cost-to-charge ratios to account for different hospital pricing policies (Pettingill and Vertrees, 1982).
4. Using both relative value units and cost-to-charge ratios (Arthur Young, 1986b).

None of these approaches is without flaws and each involves arbitrary assumptions about how overhead costs (at both the hospital and department level) are allocated to individual patients. A major constraint to more accurate costing is that nursing acuity levels and proper allocations for operating room time have not been developed.

The Health Care Financing Administration has used both the second and third approaches in calculating cost weights for DRGs. For example, in determining relative cost of DRGs using only charge information, HCFA calculated the average charge for each DRG using charge data on all hospitalized Medicare patients in 1984 and then scaled the averages so that the average charge per discharge was equal to one. Thus DRG 121 (circulatory disease with AMI) has a weight of 1.777, because the average charges for DRG 121 discharges nationally was 77.7 percent higher than the average charge across all DRGs.

Differences in Practice Patterns

Part of the difference in costs of treating patients, and in turn in the costs across hospitals, arises from physician practice patterns. There is no firmly established way of treating patients with a given condition. Some physicians may order more diagnostic tests than others, some may keep their patients in the hospital for a longer period of time, and some may make more intensive use of special care units. If physicians in some hospitals order more diagnostic tests or keep their patients longer in the hospital compared to physicians in other hospitals, then the costs of patient care will be higher in those hospitals. If practice patterns vary systematically across groups of hospitals, it follows that costs of patient care will vary across those groups. The majority of analysts who have studied differences in treatment methods across different types of hospitals have concluded that, for a given case, treatment is more resource intensive in hospitals with a large commitment to clinical education (Garg et al., 1982; Schroeder and

O'Leary, 1977; Reuben, 1984). As noted in chapter 1, the costs of the more intensive resource utilization in hospitals with a large commitment to clinical education is a major component of what has been labeled the indirect costs of clinical education.

A recent investigation of practice pattern differences analyzed the cost of treating patients in eight different DRGs by comparing hospital charge information from a sample of hospitals in four states (Cromwell, 1985). This study found that patients in major teaching hospitals (hospitals with at least 0.25 residents per bed) received more services and procedures using sophisticated technologies than patients in nonteaching hospitals did. For a given DRG, the utilization of sophisticated services (e.g., cerebral angiography) was similar in minor teaching (less than 0.25 residents per bed) and nonteaching hospitals, whereas the use of less sophisticated ancillary services was similar in both kinds of teaching hospitals. This difference in service utilization accounts for much of the difference in the costs of treating patients within a given DRG across different groups of hospitals. It also accounts for much of the difference in the costs of treating patients in hospitals in the same teaching category—a cost variation we have masked by showing only average data.

We should note that recent changes in the methods of financing hospital care as well as new control mechanisms being implemented by payors are expected to lead to a diminution in practice pattern differences across hospitals. This diminution is expected to occur both because of changes in financial incentives and because of the increased monitoring of treatment decisions by agencies external to the hospital.

Revenues

In 1986, patient revenue accounted for about 93 percent of total net hospital revenue. In general, since most patients are covered by a health insurance plan, hospitals do not receive revenues from patients directly but rather through third parties—insurance companies, employer self-administered plans, and governments. Almost 90 percent of hospital patient revenue comes through these third parties.

In chapter 2 we discussed the rules under which third parties make payments and noted how these were changing. Hospital revenue is a function of the types of insurance policies their patients hold. Payments made by some insurance plans, in particular commercial insurance plans and by self-insured plans, are related to charges, whereas payments made by other insurance plans are based on prospectively set rates. The process by which these prospective rates are set vary across plans. Relative to charges, payments are highest for private insurance plans and lowest for the Medicaid plans and the relationship between Medicare charges and payments vary significantly across hospitals.

With respect to type of hospital, public COTH hospitals admit the highest proportion of Medicaid and uninsured patients. There are few differences across the other groups of hospitals with respect to expected insurance coverage.

Control

A number of factors influence the distribution of patients among hospitals. In the past, decisions about where patients would be hospitalized and how long they would remain as inpatients were made by patients and their physicians. Unless patients were without insurance or were covered by a plan with substantial cost sharing, it is unlikely that their decision would be influenced by the relative cost of care in different hospitals. However, this laissez-faire situation has altered considerably in recent years. Many of the changes that influence the distribution of patients across hospitals have been alluded to earlier. Here we discuss some of those trends in more detail.

Capitation

Health maintenance organizations were introduced in the United States in 1929 (MacLeod and Prussin, 1973). Since 1980, however, the growth rate has accelerated, and HMOs and other capitated systems have begun to have a significant impact on where people receive hospital care. Individuals enrolled in these capitated systems do not have freedom to choose among providers; they must receive their care at hospitals where the system has made explicit contracts (except when out of the service area or in emergency conditions). While some HMOs own their own hospitals, most contract with community hospitals to provide inpatient care to enrollees.

Under a capitated plan, the delivery system assumes the risk for providing care. This means that the delivery system has strong incentives to monitor utilization, encourage the efficient use of hospital services, and use hospitals that provide services of a given quality at the lowest possible price. Since the cost of treating a given condition is higher at hospitals with extensive involvement in clinical education, HMOs have a financial incentive to contract with community or minor teaching hospitals for common procedures and to use teaching hospitals only for those services that they are uniquely qualified to render (Hoft and Glaser, 1982).

The movement to capitation has been encouraged by actions taken in both the public and private sectors. For example, under the Omnibus Budget Reconciliation Act of 1981, the Congress modified the Medicaid program's freedom-of-choice provisions to make it easier for states to enroll Medicaid recipients in capitated health care systems. The following year, TEFRA changed the way HMOs are paid in order to encourage the enrollment of Medicare beneficiaries. Private business as well as governments at all levels have implemented policies to encourage their employees to enroll in capitated systems. Enrollment in such plans has increased from 2 percent in 1980 to almost 10 percent in 1987 (Interstudy, 1988).

Preferred Provider Organizations

A recent development in the financing of health care services is the growth of preferred provider organizations, or PPOs (Gabel and Erman, 1984; de Lissovoy et al., 1987). PPOs can be organized by a traditional insurance company, by a group of providers (which will then arrange for an insurance company to market the PPO or sell its own insurance), or by a company with a self-insured health plan. The basis for determining participating providers varies across PPOs: they can be a set of providers that agree to give discounts, a set of providers identified as being the most efficient, or a set of providers that get together and form themselves into a delivery system in an attempt to assure patient volume. PPOs are sufficiently diverse that someone allegedly observed, "if you have seen one PPO, you have seen one PPO."

Preferred provider plans are designed to influence the choices of the insured population. An enrollee in a PPO usually has the option of using the preferred providers with little or no cost sharing or of using other providers at a higher cost. Consequently, it is to the financial advantage of the enrollee to use the participating providers.

Utilization Control Programs

Utilization control programs have been in place for many years. These programs are designed to encourage people to receive services in the most appropriate setting (inpatient versus outpatient), to deter unnecessary admissions (for both medical and surgical reasons) and to eliminate unnecessary days of hospitalization.

The number of formal utilization programs has been increasing over time (Gabel et al., 1987). Some of the programs are being implemented by third-party payors, while others are marketed by new companies (occasionally subsidiaries of insurance companies) directly to private employers. Utilization management firms have often developed large files of claims data, from which they develop patterns of care profiles—profiles they use in making decisions. One variant of utilization control activity is that represented by utilization and quality control peer review organizations (PROs). These organizations were established to monitor the quality and appropriateness of care provided to Medicare beneficiaries.

While early utilization control programs were considered only modestly effective, more recent programs appear to be more promising. The PROs have been credited with contributing to the decrease in Medicare admissions after PPS was implemented. An evaluation of a utilization review program, which monitored the care of employees of a private company, found that it reduced admissions by 12.3 percent and inpatient days by 8 percent (Feldstein, Wiekizer, and Wheeler, 1988).

Case Management

A new form of utilization control, case management, is becoming more prevalent. Case management can have a number of manifestations. Some Medicaid programs, for example, identify recipients who are high users of health care services and assign case managers to monitor and manage their use of health care services. Another approach is to identify patients, such as neonates, burn patients, and accident victims, who have a condition that is potentially high cost. The case manager will then work with the patients and their providers to develop a plan of care, which may include services not covered as standard services. The goal of this approach is to try to remove patients from costly settings such as hospitals and provide them with lower levels of care as quickly as possible.

Select Providers

Most third-party payors will make payments to any qualified hospital for rendering a covered service. In contrast, HMOs and other capitated systems have always had direct control over where their enrollees receive services. It is possible that third-party payors may become more restrictive in the future. For example, under regulations governing payments for heart transplants for Medicare beneficiaries, Medicare will pay only providers that meet criteria established to assure quality of service.

Cost Sharing

While cost sharing may not be viewed as a specific control technique, it may have some effect on the distribution of patients among hospitals. Cost sharing has been implemented (1) to decrease employer and government costs of providing health benefits to employed and covered populations and (2) to encourage the efficient use of hospital and medical services. If consumers who are subjected to substantial cost sharing have information on how much it will cost them to be hospitalized for a particular problem in a number of hospitals, this information may influence their choice of a hospital. Some employers are making this type of data available to their employees. Given that the cost of treating specific diseases is higher at teaching hospitals, the increased use of cost sharing may lead to a decrease in the demand for care at those hospitals.

Hospital Control

So far we have focused on how organizations other than providers and patients are changing the environment within which hospital services are provided. As outside organizations monitor hospital activities and change the rules governing patients' choices among hospitals, the providers' autonomy is reduced. Hospitals, however, are not passive agents: they can react by controlling their environment. By making decisions to add or cut services, they can influence the types of patients they will attract. By implementing management information and control systems, they can increase their efficiency. They can also advertise their services. Many hospitals are establishing their own health maintenance organization, satellite outpatient clinics, and other organizations to attract patients. Hospitals are creating special wings to provide long-term care or providing home health services in order to reduce the need for long hospital stays.

Hospitals can control, to some extent, the nature of patients admitted and the quality of care provided. Under prospective payment systems certain patients are considered profitable. This situation arises because, with few exceptions, the hospital receives a fixed payment for taking care of all patients classified into a particular DRG, even though not all of them require the same amount of resources.

It may be possible for a hospital to cut back on services or even avoid admitting patients who require more resources. Hospitals can take explicit actions to try to attract profitable patients and to discourage unprofitable patients. They might, for example, change the hours that the emergency room is open or avoid contracts with skilled nursing facilities to discourage transfers. Hospitals can also vary services to patients; under PPS, the fewer services provided to a patient, the higher the hospital's profits for that patient. There is some concern that hospitals may respond inappropriately to the incentives embedded in PPS by reducing the level and quality of care. Indeed, the more costly patients within a DRG may be at risk for an inappropriate reduction in services.

The Effect of Recent Changes on Patient Distribution

Some observers predict that changes in hospitals' external environment—particularly the prevalence of prospective payment systems, capitation, and price competition—will have some effect on the distribution of patients across categories of hospitals. There are incentives for regionalization and centralization of treatment and resources for specific conditions; for example, payment systems based on DRGs or other patient classification systems are likely to encourage the centralization of services that respond to economies of scale. Incentives for centralization should lead to a further increase in the concentration of patients with specific conditions in COTH hospitals. However, most conditions do not require sophisticated facilities and services. Consequently, to the extent that competition for patients is based on price, nonteaching hospitals and minor teaching hospitals should increase their market share.

During the early 1980s, there was debate concerning how different hospitals would fare in the new environment. Some analysts believed that teaching hospitals would be able to retain or increase their market share. They argued that "competition for patients should not be a problem for the large urban hospitals, especially those involved in teaching. The occupancy rate for firms with tertiary-care centers is maintained through referral by previous graduates, or prestige or both" (Barocci, 1981, p. 85). Others, however, were less optimistic about the future of the teaching hospital. First, teaching hospitals had trained a large number of physicians, many of whom were able to treat in minor teaching or nonteaching hospitals medical conditions that once could be treated only at academic health centers. Second, given the increasing importance of price to consumers, many believed that the less expensive nonteaching hospitals would be able to compete favorably for patients.

Between 1980 and 1986, hospital admissions fell from 34.3 million to 30.8 million, a decrease of 10 percent, while inpatient days fell from 259 million to 218 million, a decrease of almost 16 percent. However, the pattern of change in admissions and patient days differed across the four groups of hospitals. Between 1980 and 1986, admissions in COTH hospitals increased by less than 1 percent, while admissions in non-COTH teaching hospitals decreased by 9 percent. Inpatient days decreased for all groups of hospitals (16 percent), but the decrease was much larger for nonteaching than teaching hospitals (18 and 13 percent, respectively).

The result of these different patterns is that, over the period 1980–1986, COTH hospitals were also able to increase their market share; the market share of the other teaching hospitals remained constant, while that of nonteaching hospitals decreased. Table 3-5 presents the data on the distribution of admissions and patient days across the four groups of hospitals. Further analysis of the data indicate that the increase in market share was experienced by both public and private COTH hospitals. This conclusion is important, because as indicated in chapter 6, the number of people without insurance increased over this time period. If the increase in market share had been found only in public COTH hospitals, then the most logical interpretation of these results would have been that the shift was related primarily to changing levels of insurance. There are a number of possible explanations as to why the market share for teaching hospitals has increased.

First, some of the increase is accounted for by the fact that the decrease in admissions and patient days experienced over this time period was less likely to affect COTH hospitals. Some of the decrease in admissions was due to a shift of surgical cases from inpatient to

Table 3-5. Distributions of Admissions and Patient Days, by Type of Hospital, 1980–1986 (percent)

Hospital Type	1980	1981	1982	1983	1984	1985	1986
Admissions							
Major COTH	7.0	7.0	7.1	7.3	7.6	8.0	8.3
Minor COTH	12.5	12.5	12.5	12.6	12.9	13.2	13.6
Other teaching	28.2	28.2	28.2	28.3	28.4	28.5	28.6
Nonteaching	52.2	52.3	52.1	51.8	51.1	50.2	49.5
Patient Days							
Major COTH	8.4	8.3	8.4	8.6	9.0	9.5	9.7
Minor COTH	14.3	14.1	14.1	14.1	14.4	14.6	14.9
Other teaching	28.6	28.6	28.4	28.4	28.4	28.3	28.2
Nonteaching	48.7	49.0	49.1	48.9	48.2	47.6	47.2

Source: Based on data from American Hospital Association, A, 1980–86.

Note: Due to merging of data over multiple years, the number of hospitals in each category is slightly different than when characteristics for a single year are reported elsewhere in the text.

outpatient settings. We believe that a lower proportion of their surgical case loads, compared to those of other hospitals, are candidates for such a shift. Some of the decrease in admissions was attributed to a decrease in marginally necessary medical admissions. Again, because COTH hospitals treat patients who are referred to them (chapter 3) it is likely that fewer of their medical cases fall into that category.

Second, some of the increase may be a by-product of the increase in second-opinion surgery plans. As discussed above, many health plans, both public and private, require that patients who are referred for surgery get second opinions. Many of these referrals are to physicians who practice in teaching hospitals. The patient may prefer the doctor providing the second opinion and elect to receive care at the teaching hospital.

Third, teaching hospitals have been developing horizontally and vertically integrated health care delivery systems, which increase their referral bases. In addition, alternative delivery systems have frequently contracted with teaching hospitals to provide some services in order to attract patients. As health maintenance organizations and preferred provider organizations become established, however, the need for including the teaching hospital in the network, except for tertiary care services not available elsewhere, may diminish.

The final explanation for the increase is that the importance of real price competition may have been exaggerated. In spite of all the policy discussions, it is possible that price competition was simply not very strong or pervasive.

It is difficult to predict whether the pattern of admissions by hospital category will continue. On the one hand, with the spread of HMOs and PPOs and the increase in price competition, one might expect some decrease in the market share of hospitals that produce the most costly patient care services. On the other hand, because teaching hospitals tend to maintain high volumes, they may be better able to benefit from economies of scale for cases with high fixed costs and thus be able to maintain or increase market share. Finally, the search for quality may lead to an increased share of patients being admitted to COTH hospitals. The future net effect of these trends is not easily predicted.

chapter 4 | Clinical Education

Most health professionals in the United States receive a significant portion of their clinical training in hospitals. Medical students, residents, fellows, nursing students and allied health students (physical therapists, etc.) all receive some portion of their training in teaching hospitals. The clinical training of these health professionals increases the cost of the product provided by the hospital and changes its nature. Equally important is the influence of clinical training on the future of the health care system. Methods of patient care learned during clinical training are applied to clinical practice, thus affecting the cost and quality of medical care in the long run. Specialty decisions made during residency influence the future geographic and specialty distribution of physicians.

The area of clinical training most closely examined in recent years is graduate medical education, the period of formal medical education that begins after graduation from medical school and ends after the educational requirements for one or more of the medical specialty boards have been completed. The length of residency training varies from three to seven years, depending on the specialty chosen. The first year is generally referred to as the internship, and the subsequent years are the residency. Nearly all U.S. medical school students pursue graduate medical education training upon completion of medical school. Many medical school graduates from other countries also receive graduate medical education in the United States.

We have concentrated our examination of clinical training on graduate medical education for several reasons. First, the cost associated with residency education is greater than the cost for the clinical training of other health professionals, such as nurses. Second, data are available on the scope, location, and cost of graduate medical education, so we can evaluate its impact on the hospital and the changes it has undergone in response to public policy. This information is not generally available for most other programs. Third, residency training can have a major influence on the future distribution of physicians. Finally, because of the cost and distributional impact of residency training programs, public policy makers are beginning to examine the desirability of additional control over the costs, length of training, and distribution associated with residency programs.

Background

The system of graduate medical education developed slowly in the United States. In the late nineteenth century it was popular for physicians to travel to Edinburgh, Paris, or Vienna for postdoctoral training. Graduate medical education was reserved almost exclusively for the elite who studied in foreign hospitals, labs, and clinics. Unlike the United States, Europe already had large hospitals and clinics where physicians could train to develop clinical skills (Stevens, 1978). The faculty of U.S. medical schools frequently were trained in Europe under this system.

Before World War I, the most common form of clinical training in the United States was an apprenticeship with an established physician prior to medical school enrollment. Since there was no systematic postgraduate training in the United States, additional clinical experience was gained in the first years of practice. As hospitals became more accessible to practitioners, graduate medical education became increasingly important as a part of formal training for clinical experience. Initially, the demand for structured programs exceeded the supply, and entry was restricted to graduates of certain medical schools or other criteria. However, between 1880 and 1900 there was a rapid increase in the number of hospitals, and graduate medical education became available to a larger number of practitioners. Johns Hopkins, for instance, established residency training programs in the 1890s for a small number of physicians. However, residency training for physicians was rare before World War I. In fact, until 1914 graduate medical education was not a requirement for licensure as a physician in any state.

On June 11, 1910, Bulletin 4 of the Carnegie Foundation for the Advancement of Teaching, popularly known as the Flexner Report, advocated sweeping changes in medical education and research. A key recommendation was that a hospital be attached to a medical school to provide clinical training. Cutbacks in the number of medical schools

Table 4-1.   Growth in Residencies and Internships, 1930–1985

Year	Number of Hospitals Participating	Residencies or Internships Offered	Residencies or Internships Filled
1930	338	7,524	
1940	587	11,909	
1950	1,079	28,734	22,515
1960	1,307	45,333	37,562
1970	1,517	61,938	51,115
1980	1,566	70,627	62,853
1985	1,554	76,411	74,514

Source: Based on data from American Medical Association, A, 1930–86.

after the reforms generated by the Flexner Report coupled with a rapid increase in hospitals created an imbalance between the supply of residents and demand for house staff. During this period there were twice as many positions as interns and residents.

Residency Programs

Most of the growth in residency training occurred after World War II and before 1970. As shown in table 4-1, the number of hospitals participating in graduate medical education and the number of residencies offered increased substantially between 1940 and 1970, and both have remained relatively constant since 1980. Generous support from NIH after World War II provided the initial support necessary for the growth of full-time faculties at teaching hospitals. These grants were ostensibly awarded for the support of research and research training but were frequently used to support a full-time faculty (Relman, 1984b).

Foreign Medical Graduates

The United States has repeatedly used immigration and other manpower policies to affect the supply of medical graduates for residency positions and fully trained physicians. In times of perceived shortages of physicians or residents, additional foreign medical graduates (FMGs) have been allowed to train in the United States. In times of perceived surplus, admission of FMGs into the country has been more difficult.

In 1965, in response to the perceived need for more physicians, immigration statutes were revised to make it easier for FMGs to enter

Table 4-2.   Ratio of U.S. Medical School Graduates to First-Year Residency Positions, 1930–1985

Year	Ratio, Graduates to Positions	Year	Ratio, Graduates to Positions
1930	1:16	1976	1:21
1940	1:29	1977	1:24
1950	1:53	1978	1:20
1960	1:79	1979	1:20
1970	1:87	1980	1:21
1971	1:86	1981	1:18
1972	1:82	1982	1:16
1973	1:87	1983	1:15
1974	1:58	1984	1:14
1975	1:29	1985	1:15

Source: Based on data from American Medical Association, A, 1930–86.

the country for residency training and to remain after they had completed their courses of study. In this way, the pool of licensed physicians grew. When this policy began, FMGs accounted for one of every four residents; the proportion increased to one in three in the early 1970s (Ginzberg, 1982). During this same period, the federal government encouraged the growth of medical schools and the number of U.S.-trained medical students.

Immigration policy was re-examined in the mid-1970s, when projections indicated an impending surplus of physicians by 1990 (U.S. Department of Health and Human Services, 1980). The earlier programs had been so successful in attracting FMGs that, in 1976 and 1977, Congress enacted amendments to the Immigration and Nationality Act to restrict the flow of FMGs into residency training. Concern of a surplus also led to the passage of the Health Professions Educational Assistance Act in 1976 (PL 94-484), which attempted to ensure that the production of U.S. medical graduates would meet the nation's future medical needs without continued reliance on foreign manpower; it required that any FMGs entering the United States meet the same standards as American graduates.

The Demand for Residency Positions

In recent years, the number of residency positions available has not kept pace with the number of U.S. medical school graduates seeking residency positions. According to table 4-2, there is approximately the same ratio of first-year residency positions to U.S. medical school graduates in 1985 as there was in 1930. During the period from 1930 to 1970, the number of available positions per graduate increased substantially. However, since 1970 it has dropped almost every year. This decline is due primarily to the substantial increase in medical school graduates resulting from the federal health manpower policy in the 1960s. The number of students graduating from medical schools in this country is still less than the number of first-year residency positions. However, studies indicate that approximately 2,500 of these positions are considered to provide a poor educational experience by these students and that the supply of desirable positions has become almost equal to the number of U.S. graduates seeking residency positions (Stimmel and Benenson, 1979).

The Control of Residency Programs

The issue of who should control residency programs has been debated for many years without agreement. While hospitals have historically controlled residency programs (e.g., numbers trained and actual program content), there have been repeated suggestions that medical schools should have greater control of graduate medical education, since it is a continuation of the educational process. Considerable debate also concerns who should monitor overall educational standards. Individual specialty societies and residency review committees, which are generally composed exclusively of specialists from within a discipline, establish the minimum standards for each specialty. They are not, however, geared toward determining the extent to which additional specialists are actually needed.

More important, the groups that monitor the educational program have no responsibility for the financial impact of their decisions. In most organizations, control of standards and responsibility for the bottom line are vested in the same entity, whereas in medicine, they are not. Indeed, although the federal government funds much of this training, it does not have an active role in establishing standardization requirements or the number of positions available to train physicians in different disciplines. Because the Medicare prospective payment system provides substantial support to graduate medical education, the proper role of the federal government in monitoring these programs is currently being debated.

As a structured system of graduate medical education evolved, divergent interests of the various groups participating in the control process emerged and positions evolved. Before World War I, the AMA supported the control of specialty education through direct university supervision and supported the position that the university degree should be the organizing focus of graduate medical education. The AMA also wanted to establish some control over this postgraduate training and to maintain a leadership role in the field. Toward that end, they surveyed existing internships in 1912, developed the first listing of approved internships in 1914, and in 1919 developed the essentials for internship approval. By 1920, although there was no clear definition of an intern, there were criteria for approved and non-approved internships.

In 1925, the AMA took a second step and compiled a list of approved hospital residencies. In 1927, the Council on Medical Education was established to oversee residency programs and to attempt to maintain a leadership role in education; the essentials for residency training were produced, which emphasized the importance of hospital experience. By this time, the AMA had abandoned the belief that graduate medical education needed to be linked to a university and declared that it was unnecessary for hospitals providing residency training to be affiliated with a university.

Specialists supported the need for standards as early as 1917 (Stevens, 1978). The issue from the standpoint of surgeons and practitioners was not whether specialist training programs should be supervised but which organization or organizations should be responsible for developing credentials. Ophthalmology took the lead in establishing credentials and implemented the first specialty board in 1917 to certify physicians deemed to be appropriately trained in the field. Other areas of specialty training followed, and by 1987, twenty-four independent specialty boards determined the educational requirements for certification in each specialty. Each specialty society has the authority to determine the length of the program and the specific components of the training required before a physician is eligible to become board certified in that specialty. Table 4-3 shows when each specialty board was incorporated and the number of residents in each program in 1985.

In the 1940s, specialty societies became increasingly involved in providing standardized training. Committees from each specialty recommended educational standards for residency programs. These recommendations were then presented to the specialty society for final approval or revision. The committees were also responsible for approval or disapproval of programs in each hospital. In 1952, the com-

Table 4-3.   Growth of Medical Specialty Boards, 1917–1979

Medical Specialty	Year of Incorporation	Number of Residents in 1985	Percentage of Total Residents	Years of Residency Required
Opthalmology	1917	1,561	2.1	4
Otolaryngology	1924	1,094	1.5	5
Obstetrics/gynecology	1930	4,630	6.2	6
Dermatology	1932	772	1.0	4
Pediatrics	1933	6,553	8.8	3
Orthopedic surgery	1934	1,817	3.8	7
Radiology	1934	3,730	5.0	4
Psychiatry	1934	5,389	7.3	4
Neurology	1934	1,386	1.9	4
Colon and rectal surgery	1934	45	0.1	6
Urology	1935	1,057	1.4	6.5
Internal medicine	1936	17,832	23.9	3
Pathology	1936	2,488	3.5	4
Surgery	1937	8,145	10.9	5
Anesthesiology	1937	4,025	5.4	4
Plastic surgery	1937	405	0.5	5
Neurological surgery	1940	704	0.9	8
Physical medicine	1947	763	1.0	4
Preventive medicine	1948	448	0.6	4
Thoracic surgery	1948	285	0.4	7
Family practice	1969	7,276	9.8	3
Allergy/immunology	1971	276	0.4	5
Nuclear medicine	1971	191	0.3	4
Emergency medicine	1979	1,122	1.5	3

Source: Adapted from American Board of Medical Specialties, 1985.

mittees became known as residency review committees (RRC). By 1956, nearly all specialties had established RRCs. At that time, membership on the RRCs was limited to a representative of the AMA and of the specialty board; specialty societies were excluded.

In 1972, the AMA set about to establish a residency accreditation committee with broader representation than the RRCs. This change was in response to the U.S. Office of Education's criticism that the federal government had limited representation in issues regarding graduate medical education and that most issues were being controlled by the AMA. In response, a new committee, the Liaison Committee on Graduate Medical Education (LCGME), was formed composed of representatives from the AMA, the Association of American Medical Colleges, the American Board of Medical Specialties, the Council of Medical Specialty Societies, and the American Hospital Association. The federal government was a nonvoting member of the LCGME.

The Distribution of Clinical Education

Geographic Distribution

Residency positions are not distributed evenly across states. The first major academic health centers were established in large urban areas on the East Coast, and although residency education has extended beyond these cities, it is still focused in the nation's major urban centers. Table 4-4 presents the geographic distribution of residency training programs by state. Three states, New York, Pennsylvania, and California, train over 30 percent of all residents.

The distribution of residents is not always proportional to the population. New York, for example, trains almost 15 percent of the residents but has less than 10 percent of the U.S. population. Two states, Alaska and Montana, do not train any residents. Referring to residents in relation to population, the District of Columbia trains the most, at 256 per 100,000 population, and New York is second, at 61 per 100,000 population. The Northeast has the highest concentration of residents per 100,000 population, while the South and West have the lowest.

Few public policy initiatives have been specifically designed to influence the geographic distribution of residency programs. New York State recently issued a report (Report of the New York State Commission on Graduate Medical Education) that recognizes that "residency programs in New York state are disproportionately large relative to population, medical school output, and to the other states in the U.S." The commission recommended that the annual number of first-year residency positions be reduced over five years to near parity with the New York state medical school output, a reduction of approximately 30 percent. Other states are also examining their commitment to graduate medical education, given the perceived surplus of physicians, the geographic maldistribution of practicing physicians, and the costs associated with graduate medical training (New York State Commission, 1986).

Because many residents do not ultimately practice in the state

Table 4-4.   Geographical Distribution of Hospital Residents, 1985

Region and State	Number of Residents	Percentage of Total Residents	Residents per 100,000 Population
Northeast	23,038	30.92	46
Connecticut	1,532	2.06	48
Maine	156	0.21	13
Massachusetts	2,995	4.02	51
New Hampshire	160	0.21	16
New Jersey	1,942	2.61	26
New York	10,916	14.65	61
Pennsylvania	4,804	6.45	41
Rhode Island	365	0.49	38
Vermont	168	0.23	31
Southeast	10,973	14.73	27
Delaware	166	0.22	27
District of Columbia	1,603	2.15	256
Florida	1,690	2.27	15
Georgia	1,352	1.81	23
Maryland	1,949	2.62	44
North Carolina	1,600	2.15	26
South Carolina	687	0.92	21
Virginia	1,481	1.99	26
West Virginia	444	0.60	23
North Central	18,126	24.33	31
Illinois	4,049	5.43	35
Indiana	938	1.26	17
Iowa	682	0.92	24
Kansas	582	0.78	24
Michigan	3,095	4.15	34
Minnesota	1,580	2.12	38
Missouri	1,635	2.19	33
Nebraska	405	0.54	25
North Dakota	106	0.14	15
Ohio	3,777	5.07	35
South Dakota	80	0.11	11
Wisconsin	1,197	1.61	25
South	10,049	13.49	24
Alabama	847	1.14	21
Arkansas	422	0.57	18
Kentucky	721	0.97	19
Louisiana	1,370	1.84	31
Mississippi	336	0.45	13
Oklahoma	648	0.87	20
Tennessee	1,269	1.70	27
Texas	4,436	5.95	27
West	11,477	15.40	24
Alaska	0	0.00	0
Arizona	742	1.00	23
California	7,261	9.74	28
Colorado	908	1.22	28
Hawaii	353	0.47	33

Idaho	18	0.02	02
Montana	0	0.00	0
Nevada	91	0.12	10
New Mexico	252	0.34	17
Oregon	493	0.66	18
Utah	415	0.56	25
Washington	905	1.21	21
Wyoming	39	0.05	08
Territory of Puerto Rico	851	1.14	
Total	74,514	100.00	31

Source: Based on data from U.S. Bureau of the Census, 1986.

where they are trained, producing more residents does not necessarily guarantee more physicians in that state. Illinois, for example, the third largest producer of medical graduates, is thirty-third in retention of the medical personnel trained. A recent study, sponsored by the U.S. Department of Health and Human Services, reported that a variety of federal and state programs have been developed to influence the geographic distribution of health care professionals by intervening at key points in their career decision process. The most common state approaches are financial incentives for health care professionals in training to choose certain locations. Thirty-nine of the 113 state programs identified use financial incentives in the form of loans, scholarships, and grants, and require that recipients serve in areas of shortage or offer other services as alternatives to cash paybacks. Thirty-two states have programs designed to assist underserved communities in attracting physicians or to assist physicians looking for communities in which to establish a practice (U.S. Department of Health and Human Services, 1986b).

The effectiveness of programs that assist physicians in establishing and maintaining practice in underserved areas appears to depend on the level of ongoing support. The outcomes of state programs are mixed, but the results indicate that multiple strategies are the most successful in attracting and retaining physicians to shortage areas. Service-contingent programs are effective in the short run, but more permanent retention of physicians may require changes in the method of paying physicians (U.S. Department of Health and Human Services, 1986b).

Table 4-5. Residency Training, by Type of Hospital, 1986

Hospital Type	Number of Hospitals	Average Number of Residents	Percentage of Total Residents
Major COTH	119	232	45.8
Other COTH	210	96	33.4
Other teaching	859	14	19.3
Nonteaching	4,354	0	0

Source: Based on data from American Hospital Association, A, 1986.

Table 4-6. Concentration of Residency Programs, by Type of Hospital, 1986 (percent)

Hospital Type	0–5 Programs	6–10 Programs	11 Programs
Major COTH	3.36	62.19	34.45
Other COTH	26.66	64.28	9.05
Other teaching	77.23	17.57	5.20

Source: Based on data from American Hospital Association, A, 1986.

Distribution by Training Site

State medical examiners' offices, blood banks, ambulatory clinics, and mental health agencies regularly provide sites for residency training. However, over 80 percent of graduate medical education is conducted in hospitals (American Medical Association, A, 1986). Of the nearly 5,542 community hospitals in the United States in 1986, we classified 1,188 as teaching hospitals. However, the distribution is much more concentrated than this number suggests, since nearly 46 percent of all residents are trained in the 119 major COTH hospitals and 79 percent are trained in COTH hospitals (table 4-5).

The classification of hospitals into four groups ignores some of the variation among hospitals. For example, the average number of residents trained in major COTH hospitals is 232, but the range is from less than 100 to over 1,000. Scope of training, as measured by the number of residency programs offered, also varies dramatically. The proportion of hospitals having all eleven residency programs (the maximum reported to AHA), is 34.5 percent for major COTH, 9.0 percent for minor COTH, and 5.2 percent for all other teaching hospitals (table 4-6).

Data on the types of physicians trained in the different hospital categories indicate that a greater proportion of the highly specialized, procedure-oriented training programs are provided by major COTH hospitals, while primary care tends to be concentrated in other teach-

Table 4-7. Residents Trained in Each Specialty, by Type of Hospital, 1985 (percent)

Hospital Type	Radiology	Pathology	Pediatrics	General	OB/GYN	Internal Medicine	General and Family Practice
Major COTH	55.99	55.81	47.51	41.14	39.68	35.88	17.82
Other COTH	25.09	26.74	24.93	30.38	31.55	31.05	16.93
Other teaching	18.92	17.45	27.56	8.48	28.76	33.06	65.26

Source: Based on data from American Hospital Association, A, 1985.

ing hospitals (table 4-7). For example, major COTH hospitals train 56 percent of all radiology residents but only 18 percent of family practice residents. On the other hand, other teaching hospitals train only 17 percent of pathologists but 65 percent of family practice residents.

Payment Reforms and Distribution

Another issue is that the delivery site for health care is changing. Because so many of the less complex medical and surgical services are now provided on an outpatient basis, the average inpatient may be more severely ill. Therefore, hospital-based residents may not be receiving the same breadth of training as in the past. Traditionally, hospital outpatient facilities have been less willing to tolerate residents because they are slower and less efficient diagnosticians than fully trained physicians. Reimbursement systems have contributed to the bias against outpatient training, because education is generally not reimbursable in these settings.

Currently, there are efforts to encourage more graduate medical education training in ambulatory care sites. This training is especially difficult to finance in nonhospital settings, since most third-party payors will not reimburse for educational costs in these settings. Many policy makers believe that, as the health care system becomes less hospital based, it is necessary to train physicians to provide care in a variety of settings. As a result, the Congress has recently reversed earlier policy by permitting hospitals to receive Medicare payments for graduate medical education even if the training is conducted in ambulatory sites that are not hospital cost centers.

Table 4-8.   Programs and Residents on Duty 1 September 1985, by Specialty

Specialty	Programs Number	Programs Percentage	Residents Number	Residents Percentage
Allergy and immunology	87	1.8	276	0.4
Anesthesiology	165	3.4	4,025	5.4
Colon and rectal surgery	28	0.6	45	0.1
Dermatology	97	2.0	745	1.0
Dermatopathology	24	0.5	27	*
Emergency medicine	68	1.4	1,122	1.5
Family practice	385	8.0	7,276	9.8
Internal medicine	442	9.2	17,832	23.9
Neurological surgery	92	1.9	704	0.9
Neurology	123	2.6	1,386	1.9
Nuclear medicine	91	1.9	191	0.3
Obstetrics/gynecology	292	6.1	4,630	6.2
Ophthalmology	142	3.0	1,561	2.1
Orthopedic surgery	168	3.5	2,817	3.8
Otolaryngology	107	2.2	1,094	1.5
Pathology	261	5.4	2,358	3.2
Blood banking	34	0.7	32	*
Forensic pathology	39	0.8	49	0.1
Hematology	6	0.1	8	*
Neuropathology	58	1.2	41	0.1
Pediatrics	236	4.9	6,088	8.2
Pediatric cardiology	46	1.0	140	0.2
Neonatal and perinatal	91	1.9	325	0.4
Physical medicine and rehabilitation	71	1.5	763	1.0
Plastic surgery	101	2.1	405	0.5
Preventive medicine,				
General	26	0.5	196	0.3
Aerospace	3	0.1	62	0.1
Occupational	26	0.5	106	0.1
Public health	9	0.2	26	*
General and public health combined	7	0.1	58	0.1
Psychiatry	211	4.4	4,809	6.5
Child psychiatry	128	2.7	580	0.8
Radiology, diagnostic	211	4.4	3,132	4.2
Radiology, diagnostic, nuclear	47	1.0	74	0.1
Radiology, therapeutic	96	2.0	524	0.7
Surgery	306	6.4	8,070	10.8
Pediatric	17	0.4	24	*
Vascular	38	0.8	51	0.1
Thoracic	96	2.0	285	0.4

Urology	133	2.8	1,057	1.4
Transitional year	191	4.0	1,520	2.0
Total	4,799	100.0	74,515	100.0

Source: Adapted from American Medical Association, C, 1986/87.
Note: Programs in the recently accredited pediatric subspecialties of endocrinology, hematooncology, and nephrology are not included in this table.
*Less than 0.1 percent.

Specialty Distribution

Medical school graduates can choose among forty different types of approved residency programs. Table 4-8 lists the number of programs offered by each specialty and the number of residents training in each area in 1985. Over 70 percent of residents are trained in seven specialties: anesthesiology, family practice, internal medicine, obstetrics and gynecology, pediatrics, psychiatry, and surgery.

The scope of residency programs offered and the size of each training program are determined primarily by the sponsoring institution, which initiates the process to add, delete, expand, or reduce the size of a program. A major criticism of the current system is that it has not responded to numerous studies that have projected an imbalance between supply and need in certain specialties (U.S. Department of Health and Human Services, 1980; Petersdorf, 1985). The 1980 *Graduate Medical Education National Advisory Committee Report* calculated that the 1990 supply of physicians would fall into three categories by specialty—oversupply, balanced supply, and undersupply. This and other projections have repeatedly called for an increase in the number of primary care physicians trained and a reduction in the production of specialists and subspecialists.

Table 4-9 shows that, in spite of the findings of the report, the number of positions offered in areas of primary care relative to other specialties has not increased significantly from 1980 to 1985. There has been no systematic reduction in the number of positions offered in specialties judged to be in excess supply, nor has there been a systematic increase in specialties judged to be in undersupply.

Numerous state programs have been developed to influence physician's decisions concerning specialty choice (U.S. Department of

Table 4-9.   Change in Number of Residents, by Specialty, 1980–1985

Specialty	Number of Residents 1980	Number of Residents 1985	Percentage Change
Allergy and immunology	192	276	43.75
Anesthesiology	2,490	4,025	61.65
Colon and rectal surgery	37	45	21.62
Dermatology	755	745	−1.32
Dermatopathology	30	27	−10.00
Emergency medicine	0	1,122	
Family practice	6,344	7,276	14.69
Internal medicine	15,964	17,832	11.70
Neurological surgery	511	704	37.77
Neurology	1,114	1,386	24.42
Nuclear medicine	176	191	8.52
Obstetrics/gynecology	4,221	4,630	9.69
Ophthalmology	1,480	1,561	5.47
Orthopedic surgery	2,418	2,817	16.50
Otolaryngology	923	1,094	18.53
Pathology	2,283	2,488	8.98
Pediatrics	5,303	6,553	23.54
Physical medicine	492	763	55.08
Plastic surgery	367	405	10.35
Preventive medicine	284	448	57.75
Psychiatry	4,337	5,389	24.26
Radiology, diagnostic	2,814	3,206	13.93
Radiology, therapeutic	288	524	81.94
Surgery	7,821	8,145	4.14
Thoracic surgery	256	285	11.33
Urology	917	1,057	15.27
Transitional year	1,407	1,520	8.03
Total	63,224	74,514	17.86

Source: Based on data from American Medical Association, A, 1980–86.

Health and Human Services, 1986). Many programs are designed to choose medical school applicants predisposed to rural practice or primary care. Others attempt to affect experiences during the educational process through a support of primary care residencies, preceptorships, and grants for research in primary care. Some states have funded public medical schools, whose graduates are more likely to enter primary care in underserved areas than graduates of private medical schools (Otis, Graham, and Thacker, 1975). Several states have encouraged curriculum changes to influence specialty choice by providing alternatives to traditional hospital-based medical education. These include programs such as the Area Health Education Centers program, an effort to support training in remote practice sites and to provide continuing education and support to practicing physicians.

Foreign Medical Graduates

The training of foreign medical graduates addresses issues of both geographic and specialty distribution. There were 12,509 U.S. and foreign-born foreign medical graduates being trained in the United States in 1985, representing 16.8 percent of all residents being trained at that time (American Medical Association, A, 1985). The majority of FMGs are trained in a few states (table 4-10), and even within these states they tend to be concentrated in specific areas. New York State trains over 31 percent of all FMGs, accounting for nearly 28 percent of the residents being trained in that state. In 1984, 78.9 percent of the state's FMGs were located in New York City, with over 50 percent being trained in two boroughs, Brooklyn, 29.7 percent, and Manhattan 20.8 percent (New York State Commission on Graduate Medical Education, 1986).

Foreign medical graduates are also distributed unevenly across specialties. As a percentage of all residents, FMGs tend to be concentrated in psychiatry, pediatrics, physical medicine and rehabilitation, pathology and nuclear medicine. In each of these specialties, nearly 30 percent of all trainees are FMGs. Any specific public policy that focuses on FMGs would have a very localized effect, both regionally and across specialties.

Public policy for financing graduate medical education has recently singled out foreign-born foreign medical graduates. The number of foreign medical graduates has decreased significantly in the past six years, primarily due to amendments to the Immigration and Nationality Act. Beginning in 1978, alien foreign medical graduates have been required to demonstrate competency in English and to pass a visa-qualifying exam prior to entering a U.S. residency program (American Medical Association, C, 1978). In 1984, the Educational Commission for Foreign Medical Graduates began administering a new, more stringent examination that foreign medical school graduates must pass be-

Table 4-10. Geographic Concentration of Foreign Medical Graduates, 1985

| State | Foreign Medical Graduates | |
	Number	Percentage
New York	3,948	31.56
New Jersey	1,081	8.64
Pennsylvania	759	6.07
Illinois	984	7.87
California	595	4.76
All others	5,142	41.11

Source: Adapted from American Medical Association, A, 1985.

fore entering residency training in the United States. In the first year of the test, only 3.8 percent of U.S.-born FMGs and 17.4 percent of foreign-born FMGs passed (Iglehart, 1985a).

The Cost of Clinical Education

Training residents, nurses, medical students, and allied health professionals may increase the total cost to the institution that provides the training. Most empirical studies have examined the influence of residency programs on hospital costs and ignored the effect of nurses, medical students, and allied health trainees. In this section, we examine the costs associated with residency programs and then discuss the impact of other clinical training programs on costs for hospitals and other providers.

Most studies agree that the presence of clinical education programs increases hospital costs (Hadley, 1983b). Major COTH hospitals are more than twice as expensive as nonteaching hospitals. This does not mean, however, that all of the cost differential is attributable to clinical education. Numerous studies have tried to identify the factors that contribute to the cost differential between teaching and nonteaching hospitals and to determine how much of the difference is attributable to teaching and other factors (see chapter 1).

There is no consensus on the amount by which education increases costs in these institutions once factors such as case mix, input prices, and location are considered. This is due primarily to the difficulty of separating the costs of jointly produced services—education, patient care, and research. Since cost allocation among these services is somewhat arbitrary, any estimate of the cost of education will be imprecise.

While recognizing the difficulties associated with separating the cost of clinical education from other services, economists, accountants, clinicians, and hospital administrators have still attempted to identify the cost of clinical education. To identify the cost of graduate medical education, it has become standard to disaggregate cost into direct and indirect costs.

Direct Costs

Direct costs are easily defined and can be determined from standard accounting records of the hospital. The direct costs of graduate medical education include residents' stipends and fringe benefits, program administration (e.g., administrative salaries, office space, teaching materials, and space allocated specifically for teaching), salaries paid to teaching physicians, and any overhead costs. Direct costs, using Medicare's definition of allowable costs, were approximately $3 billion in 1985.

Residents' stipends and fringe benefits represent almost half of total direct education costs. Most of the real growth in residents' stipends occurred prior to 1970; since then, growth has only kept pace with inflation. Table 4-11 shows that, while the salaries of first-year residents increased from $8,115 to $21,776 during the period from 1970 to 1986, salaries in constant dollars actually declined from $8,743 to $8,315.

Indirect Costs

The indirect costs of medical education are not as easily defined as direct costs. They include the additional patient care costs incurred because the hospital is engaged in clinical training programs and because residents are directly involved in patient care. One major source of increased costs is greater use of ancillary services in patient care. In addition, clinical training of residents puts extra demands on physicians and other hospital personnel. The presence of nursing, allied health professionals, and medical students engaged in clinical training is also believed to increase indirect costs, although no systematic studies have been conducted that quantify the magnitude of these costs.

Most of the research into the higher cost of teaching hospitals concerns the determination of indirect costs. Early attempts to identify indirect costs were largely descriptive and limited by the availability of data; typically, they relied on a survey of one hospital or a

Table 4-11.   Average First-Year House Staff Stipends, 1940–1986

Year	Current Dollars	Constant 1972 Dollars
1940	615	1,835
1950	900	1,564
1960	2,395	3,383
1965	3,797	5,035
1970	8,115	8,743
1975	11,685	9,083
1980	16,017	8,132
1981	17,301	7,958
1982	18,910	8,196
1983	19,868	8,343
1984	20,808	8,381
1985	21,241	8,260
1986	21,766	8,315

Sources: Based on data from American Medical Association, B; C.

comparison of one teaching and one nonteaching hospital. More recent studies can be grouped into two categories: comparisons of ancillary service use and analyses of hospital cost functions.

Ancillary Use as a Measure of Indirect Costs   Table 4-12 summarizes some of the literature that addresses the issue of greater ancillary use in the teaching hospital. Increases in ancillary use attributed to education vary widely, a result that is probably caused by the diversity of methods employed to detect the differences. These studies used different methods to control for variations in case mix and other factors, which might explain differences in ancillary use.

Busby, Leming, and Olson (1972) reviewed program cost allocation in a university medical center and community hospitals. They found that educational costs included 90 percent more laboratory tests, 95 percent more X-rays, and 25 percent more electrocardiograms in teaching hospitals than in community hospitals. In a comparison of a university teaching hospital and a proprietary hospital, Schroeder and O'Leary (1977) determined that 56 percent of the difference in average billing between teaching and nonteaching hospitals could be attributed to use of diagnostic services. Garg, Elkhatib, and Kleinberg (1983) asked residents to categorize tests they ordered for 199 medical patients to determine which were for teaching purposes. Eleven percent of the tests, representing 10 percent of the ancillary charges, were for education. Other studies have compared ancillary

Table 4-12.   Increased Ancillary Usage in Teaching Hospitals, Results of Four Studies

Study	Result
Busby, Leming, and Olson, 1972	90% more laboratory tests, 95% more X-rays, and 25% more electrocardiograms in teaching hospital
Garg, Elkhatib, and Kleinberg, 1983	10% of ancillary charges attributable to education; 14% more ancillary charges on teaching floor
Martz and Ptakowski, 1978	60% more ancillary services on teaching floor
Schroeder and O'Leary, 1977	56% more diagnostic services in a teaching hospital

service charges on a teaching and nonteaching floor in the same hospital. Martz and Ptakowski (1978) found that the teaching floor had charges 1.6 times greater than the nonteaching floor, due primarily to a greater use of laboratory services. Garg, Elkhatib, and Kleinberg, controlling for patient diagnosis and attending physician, found a 14 percent increase in total charges on the teaching floor.

Although these studies reviewed the differences in ancillary usage between teaching and nonteaching units, they did not give any indication of the magnitude of the effect on hospital costs. The marginal cost of an additional test is less than the average cost. As a result, an increase in ancillary costs may not have a significant impact on hospital costs.

Interns and Residents per Bed as a Measure of Indirect Costs   Most recent studies have used the ratio of interns and residents per bed as a proxy for teaching intensity. The results of four studies, presented in table 4-13, suggest that for each resident per ten hospital beds, hospital costs increase by 4.1 to 10.5 percent. In other words, a thousand-bed hospital with 200 residents is expected to have higher costs per discharge (between 8.2 and 21.0 percent) than a similar hospital without residents, depending on which results are used. (It is not surprising that empirical results differ with model specification and the quality of the data.)

Analysis by Anderson and Lave (1986) demonstrated that parameter estimates for the ratio of interns and residents per bed are highly dependent on the other variables included in the equation (table 4-14). The addition or deletion of variables unrelated to residency education, such as size of the urban area, can influence the estimated

Table 4-13. Indirect Costs Associated with Residents, Results of Three Studies

Study	Percentage of Cost per Ten Beds
Pettingill and Vertrees, 1982	5.69
Anderson and Lave, 1986	4.7 to 8.1[a]
Arthur Young, 1986a,b,c	4.1 to 10.5[a]

[a]Dependent on model.

costs associated with graduate medical education. They estimated a series of equations by sequentially entering variables forming a more complete specification.

The first model uses four independent variables: log of the number of interns and residents per bed, log of the hospital wage index, log of case mix index, and whether the hospital was located in an urban area (1.0 if yes, 0 otherwise). These are the four variables initially used in the Medicare prospective payment system. The second model added the log of the number of beds, a measure of hospital economy of scale. Model three, which added an adjustment for the size of the metropolitan area where the hospital was located, replicated the specification orginally used by HCFA to estimate the indirect costs of medical education. Model four replaced the urban-rural variable with a more refined measure of geographic location. Model five incorporated a measure of the level of care for low-income patients, and model six included the percentage of the population urbanized.

With the inclusion of each additional factor, the parameter estimate of the interns and residents per bed variable was reduced. The study showed that the inclusion of two variables, number of beds and the more descriptive location variables, significantly affected the magnitude of the coefficient of interns and residents per bed. Thus results indicate that estimation of the indirect costs of graduate medical education is highly dependent on other variables entered into the regression model. According to this study, these additional variables reduced the estimation of cost of training from 8.1 to 4.7 percent.

Hospital and Physician Costs

A recurrent criticism of the methodologies used to estimate hospital cost functions is that they tend to overestimate the difference between teaching and nonteaching hospitals (Lave and Lave 1978; Sloan, Feldman, and Steinwald, 1983; Hosek, 1979). Theoretically, the dependent cost variable should include payments for all hospital inputs, including

Table 4-14. Factors Affecting Medicare Operating Costs per Admission, 1981

Variable	(1)	(2)	(3)[a]	(4)	(5)	(6)
R^2	.67	.70	.71	.71	.72	.72
Intercept	7.53	7.02	7.02	7.00	6.98	6.98
Interns and residents per bed	.81 (.05)	.56 (.05)	.52 (.105)	.51 (.04)	.47 (.04)	.47 (.04)
Wage index	1.16 (.03)	1.16 (.03)	1.00 (.03)	.96 (.03)	1.08 (.04)	.88 (.03)
Case mix index	1.51 (.04)	1.01 (.04)	1.05 (.04)	1.06 (.04)	.93 (.03)	1.07 (.04)
Beds		.12 (.004)	.12 (.004)	.12 (.004)	.12 (.004)	.11 (.004)
Urban (rural excluded)	.11 (.01)	.03 (.01)				
MSA_1[b]				−.004* (.01)		
MSA_2[b]				.02 (.01)		
MSA_3[b]				.02 (.01)		
MSA_A[c]				.02* (.03)	.02* (.03)	−.05* (.03)
MSA_B[c]				.002* (.01)	* (.00)	−.03* (.01)
MSA_C[c]				.024 (.01)	.025 (.012)	−.004* (.013)
MSA_D[c]				.038 (.014)	.044 (.013)	.01 (.01)
MSA_E[c]				.09 (.01)	.10 (.012)	.06 (.01)
MSA_F[c]				.17 (.01)	.17 (.01)	.12 (.02)
% population Medicaid, no pay					.19 (.03)	
% population urbanized						.001 (.0001)

Source: Anderson and Lave, 1986. Reprinted by permission.

Note: Standard errors in parentheses. Coefficients significant at .99 confidence level.

[a]This regression has the same specification as HCFA used to estimate the indirect costs. Our regression coefficients, however, are not exactly the same as those found by HCFA.

[b]MSA_1, MSA_2, and MSA_3 represent MSAs of <250,000, between 250,000 and 1 million, and 1 million, respectively.

[c]MSA_A through MSA_F represent MSAs of these populations: 100,000; 100,000 to 250,000; 250,000 to 500,000; 500,000 to 999,000; 1 million to 2.5 million; and 2.5 million, respectively.

*Statistically insignificant.

physician services. However, due to data limitations, payments made to physicians are frequently not available. This omitted variable may vary systematically with a hospital's teaching status, since typically a greater percentage of the physicians in a teaching hospital are salaried employees. Consequently, analyses of costs that exclude physician payments may produce misleading results.

A recurrent controversy in evaluating the costs of graduate medical education is the possible extent of an offset effect; that is, how much the services provided by interns and residents substitute for the services provided by hospital personnel and attending physicians, thereby defraying some costs of patient care (Jones, 1984). Residents have a dual role in the hospital; they provide medical services while simultaneously learning through on-the-job training. The extent to which students substitute for more experienced and more expensive medical personnel directly affects the incremental costs of residency training. Analyzing the incremental cost of residency education is complicated, since residents can substitute for hospital personnel as well as for physicians. In most studies of substitution of residents for other medical personnel, there was limited data on the role residents play in providing physician services.

Hosek and Massel (1976) examined the effect of teaching on direct costs in radiology departments in ninety general medical and surgical Veterans Administration (VA) hospitals in 1973. They found that, in radiology departments, direct costs for salaries of house physicians and nurses, supplies, and purchased services were lower for twenty-two diagnostic procedures in departments with residents. They suggested that these savings reflected the substitution of students for physicians and other resources. It is important to consider, however, that these results may not be generalizable to other settings or specialties. First, the VA system differs from non-VA hospitals in many respects. Further, residents in radiology are not directly involved in patient care. They perform tests but are not responsible for ordering the tests.

A 1973 study estimated the net cost to Hartford Hospital of discontinuing its teaching programs while maintaining comparable patient care services. It found that the total cost to the hospital would be slightly higher without teaching programs, because more highly paid personnel would have to be paid to provide the same services. It also found that the total cost of care, reflecting additional physician charges to patients, would be substantially higher. It concluded that physician and hospital costs would not decrease, because the cost of paying practicing physicians to provide the medical care previously provided by residents would more than offset the savings associated with terminating the teaching programs. The costs of nursing and allied health education were not balanced by the services these students provided, but they were covered by the value of medical staff services. This study focused only on direct costs and did not consider indirect costs.

A study of forty-five hospitals conducted by Arthur Young (1987) found that interns and residents substituted for attending physicians and other health care personnel. There were significant differences in substitution patterns among the different types of teaching hospitals, with the greatest degree of substitution found in major teaching hospitals. The results suggest that the skill levels of residents, nurses, and other labor resources are highest at major teaching hospitals. The results also suggest that residents, in general, can and do perform many patient care duties typically performed by attending physicians and that in major teaching hospitals there is greater flexibility in mixing labor input to produce a given amount of patient care.

Cost function analyses generate similar conclusions. Two studies using Medicaid data to examine the effect of teaching on hospital costs specifically included payments to physicians. One study (Neu, 1976) compared the costs of all Medicaid patients in five New Mexico hospitals—one major university-affiliated teaching hospital and four with little or no teaching activity. The study indicated that the teaching hospital had a significantly lower likelihood of surgery, higher utilization of intensive care units and laboratory tests, and lower payment for X-ray. The study also found that physician payments for separately billed professional services were 33 percent lower on average in the teaching hospital. More recently, Cameron (1985) compared costs of California Medicaid patients in acute care settings, controlling for patient case mix and physician compensation. For this study, hospitals were separated into four categories: (1) university, (2) major teaching, (3) minor teaching, and (4) nonteaching. He found that cost differentials were reduced when physician costs were included (table 4-15).

Cost of Allied Health Education

The factors contributing to the cost of educating students in nursing and allied health professions are similar to those discussed in the previous section. A major difficulty in determining direct costs is that, except for hospital-based nursing programs financed through Medicare, there is no standardized system of accounting for the costs of training these students in the hospital. Thus the data is insufficient to

Table 4-15.   Cost Comparisons by Type of Hospital, Using California Medicaid Data

Hospital Type	Hospital Direct Cost (dollars)	Percentage of Nonteaching	Full Physician Cost (dollars)	Percentage of Nonteaching	Combined Hospital and Physician Cost (dollars)	Percentage of Nonteaching
University	1,679	207	361	110	2,040	180
Major teaching	1,097	135	244	74	1,341	118
Minor teaching	968	119	322	99	1,290	114
Nonteaching	809	100	326	100	1,135	100

Source: Adapted from Cameron, 1985.

calculate direct costs for nursing and allied health professions programs (Gonyea, 1980).

Much of the literature on the indirect costs of the education of nurses and allied health professionals address the issue through cost-benefit analyses. Keim and Carney (1975) performed a cost analysis of the clinical portions of several formal education programs. They calculated program costs by estimating the resources used (personnel time, space, equipment, supplies, etc.) and compared these to the revenues expected from the production of hospital services. They concluded that there is no net personnel cost to the hospital in operating allied health education programs except possibly for physician assistant programs. We found one study that calculated the cost per educational program in a single medical center (Smith, 1975). His estimates of net costs for specific programs ranged from $909 to $4,704 in 1972–73.

Financing Clinical Education

Revenues associated with graduate medical education are difficult to estimate precisely. Hospitals, medical schools, and faculty practice plans have complex financial arrangements, which make the determination of the sources of revenues to finance graduate medical education extremely difficult to calculate (chapter 2).

Residency Positions

Table 4-16 shows the sources of funding for residents' stipends in 1977 and 1984. The principal source was patient care revenue. For all COTH hospitals, patient care revenues supported 77 percent of resi-

Table 4-16.   Sources of Funding for House Staff Stipends, 1977 and 1984 (percent)

Funding Source	Study 1, 1977 (252)[a]	Study 2, 1984 (280)[a]	Study 3, 1977 (432)[a]	Study 4, 1984 (418)[a]
Patient revenue and general operations	77	82	66	73
Medical school/ university funds	2	2	1	2
Government	14	9	29	24
Municipal	7	1	15	9
State	5	5	0	0
Federal	2	3	14	15
Other	7	7	5	1

Sources: Council of Teaching Hospitals, A, 1984; Council of Teaching Hospitals, 1987; Schleiter and Tarlov, 1985; Tarlov et al., 1979.
[a]Number of hospitals in sample.

dents' stipends in 1977, increasing to 82 percent in 1984. For internal medicine residency programs, the percentage of residency stipends funded through patient care revenues increased from 66 to 73 percent during this same time period. Government programs were the next largest source of funds, especially for internal medicine programs, which benefited from programs promoting primary care.

Patient Care Services

Chapter 2 states that approximately 90 percent of the average hospital's revenues are derived from patient care activities. Earlier in this chapter, we showed that a large proportion of the direct cost of resident education is supported by patient care services, and it is expected that nearly all indirect costs are covered by patient care services. It is appropriate, therefore, to begin the discussion of the financing of clinical education with patient care services. Since most empirical work has involved the Medicare program, we begin with a discussion of that program.

Medicare Financing

Direct Costs   When the Medicare program started in 1966, graduate medical education was funded implicitly through patient care revenues to the hospital. The direct costs of the education, salaries, and fringe benefits of residents and faculty physicians and all associated administrative costs were reimbursed as allowable Medicare costs. Although there was some debate at the outset concerning the appropriateness of reimbursing education costs through Medicare payments for patient care, this provision was made as an interim measure, with the intent that a more permanent policy would be established (Somers and Somers, 1967; Fruen and Korper, 1981; Hadley, 1982; Aiken and Bays, 1984). Funding for the direct costs of graduate medical education is still provided via this interim measure.

The direct costs associated with graduate medical education first became an explicit issue under the Section 223 Program, which was designed to identify high-cost hospitals and to limit payment to an appropriate level. When Section 223 regulations were first published, they established per diem limits on routine patient care costs for hospitals. Limits were set by comparing a hospital's costs with the costs of peer hospitals. Teaching was not a factor in determining peer grouping. Routine per diem costs exceeding the established limits were considered unreasonable and therefore not reimbursable by Medicare.

Analysis suggested that teaching hospitals were disproportionately affected by Section 223 limits, because their direct teaching costs were included in the calculation of routine costs. Confronted with a choice of whether they should pay for clinical education, federal regulators decided that teaching hospitals were just as efficient as nonteaching hospitals and that an adjustment in the limits for direct costs was appropriate. To equalize the adverse impact of Section 223 regulations on all types of hospitals, teaching hospitals were permitted to apply for an adjustment on an annual basis. In the first few years of Section 223 regulations, applications for adjustments by teaching hospitals to exclude their teaching cost from cost comparisons were so common that the regulations were changed in 1979 to automatically exclude direct medical education costs from the calculations of routine patient care costs.

This automatic exception, or pass through, of direct education costs was continued by all subsequent Section 223 regulations, incorporated in the Tax Equity and Fiscal Responsibility Act of 1982 (TEFRA), and adopted as part of the prospective payment legislation in 1983. In 1987, the prospective payment system provided approximately $1 billion for direct medical education costs via the pass through. These funds are in addition to the hospital's DRG payments for patient care.

Indirect Costs Improved methodology along with budgetary pressures allowed federal policy makers to consider reducing Section

223 limits. However, analysis indicated that any significant reduction would cause financial hardship for many hospitals, particularly teaching hospitals with large educational programs. Even with the pass through, teaching hospitals were still the most likely to be penalized by the Section 223 limitation. To address this issue, a number of methods to adjust Medicare payments to account for the indirect costs associated with graduate medical education were considered.

Some of the simpler approaches, such as creating a separate category for teaching hospitals, ignored the diversity of commitment to graduate medical education among teaching hospitals. After considerable deliberation, the Medicare program chose to use a continuous adjustment procedure for graduate medical education, based on ratio of residents per bed (Pettingill and Vertrees, 1982). Statistical analysis indicated that, after adjusting for bed size, location, and area wages, costs at teaching hospitals still exceeded those of nonteaching hospitals (Lave, 1985). In order to determine an appropriate adjustment factor, HCFA estimated a hospital cost function (Pettingill and Vertrees, 1982) and found that for each resident per ten beds, the Section 223 limit should increase by 5.69 percent. The indirect teaching adjustment was continued in all subsequent Section 223 regulations and in the TEFRA legislation.

When Congress began debating the prospective payment system in 1983, the Congressional Budget Office presented data that indicated that teaching hospitals could potentially lose 7 percent of Medicare revenues they would have received under TEFRA regulations if a DRG-based prospective payment system were implemented (Newhouse, 1983). According to these calculations, 71 percent of all teaching hospitals would be worse off, and as a result a political compromise was developed to double the statistically derived estimate in order to equalize the expected financial impact across all hospitals (Iglehart, 1985b).

The published reasons cited for doubling the adjustment were the lack of a severity-of-illness measure. The Senate Finance Committee report (U.S. Senate, 1983) makes it clear that the doubling of the adjustment for indirect teaching was intended to pay for more than graduate medical education. "This adjustment is provided in the light of doubts . . . about the ability of the DRG Case Classification System to account fully for factors such as severity of illness. . . . The adjustment for indirect medical education costs is only a proxy to account for a number of factors which may legitimately increase costs in teaching hospitals" (p. 52). Thus, under the original specifications for PPS, for each resident per 10 beds, the hospital received an additional 11.59

percent of the prospectively set DRG price. The magnitude of this payment can be very large for some hospitals. A hospital with 1,000 beds and 300 residents, for example, now receives an additional 34.77 percent in payment for each Medicare discharge from this indirect factor. In 1986, the adjustment factor was reduced from 11.59 percent to 8.71 percent, based on a revised statistical estimate of the magnitude of indirect costs (Sheingold, 1988). It has been reduced slightly in subsequent years. Payments for indirect medical education in the Medicare program are approximately $2 billion a year.

Medicaid Programs

States have adopted a variety of methods to pay for the costs of clinical education (Hadley, 1983a; Laudicina, 1985). The most common methods are peer grouping, which includes teaching status as one of the factors in determining the hospital's classification, trending forward a hospital's own costs, and maintaining cost-based reimbursement. All three of these systems allow teaching hospitals to recover some of the direct and indirect costs of clinical education.

Private Sector

Blue Cross and commercial insurers that use cost-based or charge-based reimbursement implicitly or explicitly include an allowance for the direct and indirect costs of clinical education. PPOs, HMOs, and other alternative delivery systems that negotiate hospital payment rates generally are reluctant to pay for clinical education explicitly; however, they tend to pay higher rates to teaching hospitals for differences in quality of care or access to specialized services available only in teaching hospitals.

Federal Grant Programs

Most early federal support of clinical education was through the National Institute of Health. By supporting biomedical research, the federal government began supporting clinical education indirectly, as funds were used to sponsor residents and other trainees involved in research projects. The Health Education Professions Educational Assistance Act (PL 14-484) promoted education in primary care specialties by requiring medical schools that wanted to qualify for the grant to graduate a certain percentage of students who would pursue residencies in primary care. Subsequent legislation established grant programs to support specific residency programs, such as family practice. Grants to these residency programs became as large as $250 million a year in the 1970s.

State Promotion of Specific Residency Programs

State funding has also been used to encourage change in the geographic or specialty distribution of medical professionals. State appropriations for graduate training in medical education have been provided to increase the number of physicians in underserved rural areas and to increase the number of primary care physicians.

Financing Teaching Physicians

Most of the revenues used to finance teaching physicians are generated from patient care funds. Because the methods of compensating teaching physicians are so diverse, precise estimates of the sources of funding are nearly impossible to obtain in specific hospitals, and even more difficult to aggregate across hospitals.

Developing appropriate methods to finance teaching physicians has been especially controversial in the Medicare program. The issue centers around alleged double billing by teaching physicians, who receive a salary under Medicare Part A for training residents and a fee under Medicare Part B for providing patient care. Medicare rules allow a teaching physician to bill a patient if certain criteria are met, including providing personal and identifiable services to the patient (IL-372). In this case, the physician is allowed to bill under Part B but should not charge for any of the time spent training residents under Part A. It is clearly difficult for the physician to monitor time spent and even more difficult for the government to monitor each teaching physician. Despite repeated attempts to make the legislation and implementing regulations more rational, the inherent difficulty of separating a physician's time when two services are being performed simultaneously makes the implementation of any regulation extremely difficult.

Payment Reforms

Recent payment reforms have caused a reduction in the hospital length of stay by almost two days (Davis et al., 1985). This may in turn change the educational process dramatically. Shorter lengths of stay allow less time for clinical training during each hospitalization. In the past, residents provided services through the entire course of treatment. Now, the resident who treats the patient in the hospital may not be involved in the preparation for the hospitalization, which frequently includes a battery of preadmission tests and the diagnosis and determination of the treatment regimen. In addition, patients now are discharged earlier in their illness or disease cycle. If the patient returns on an outpatient basis for follow-up treatment, a different resident may be assigned to provide care. Consequently, residents may no longer be involved in the entire continuum of care; the reduced length of stay may therefore have a negative effect on the quality and breadth of resident education.

Financing Allied Health Education

Nursing and allied health training programs charge their students tuition to cover a portion of the direct costs of their programs. As a result, the programs appear to be largely self-supporting. Medicare and most other third-party payors usually recognize the direct costs of nursing and allied health professions programs as reimbursable costs. To the extent that these programs incur any indirect costs during their clinical training, these costs are financed implicitly by patient care revenues.

The Control of Graduate Medical Education

The control of graduate medical education, in terms of the quality, volume, and specialty distribution, is complex because of the multiple individuals involved in the process and the distinct agendas of each participant. Controls began in an era when graduate medical education was unstructured and evolved primarily in response to the agendas of various interest groups. Consequently, the current system of control lacks a coherent framework (Stevens, 1978). Especially important is the absence of a link between the financing of the programs and their control. The major financing sources do not participate in decisions about type of program or program content.

While the present system of controls has evolved slowly, the central players and their roles have remained largely unchanged over the past six decades. Graduate medical education is controlled primarily by seven groups: (1) the American Medical Association, (2) the American Hospital Association, (3) the Association of American Medical Colleges, (4) the American Board of Medical Specialties, (5) the Council of Medical Specialty Societies, (6) federal agencies, and (7) hospitals. Representatives from these groups form various committees that control graduate medical education through program accreditation, specialty certification, and the determination of the structure and size of education programs. The structure, size, and quality of graduate medical education programs are influenced, at least in part, by all of the participants. No one group has primary responsibility.

Determinations of the scope, size, and quality of residency programs begin at the hospital level. Within the hospital, many participants may influence the types of programs offered. Hospital administrators often determine number of residents, based on what is required to fulfill the hospitals' patient care needs. Medical school deans have a strong interest in the content and quality of residency programs, since residents frequently function as teachers for medical students. Hospital program directors generally have the basic responsibility for the quality of graduate medical education. Clinical faculty associated with the medical school frequently have influence over the number of residents in their department and the content of the program. These physicians are most influential when they are part of a faculty practice plan that provides financial support for the residency program.

Accreditation Council for Graduate Medical Education

Residency programs must be accredited; residency accreditation is the responsibility of the Accreditation Council for Graduate Medical Education (ACGME), which is composed of representatives from professional organizations. The federal government names a representative to serve as a nonvoting member, and the council chooses one member from the public. The ACGME has final authority to accredit graduate medical education programs. The group can delegate this authority to the residency review committees (RRCs) on a time-limited basis, subject to monitoring and periodic review.

Residency Review Committees

Residency review committees play a major role in residency program accreditation. Following guidelines established by the ACGME, the

RRCs establish specific requirements for program accreditation, which are tailored to each specialty. These are subject to review and recommendation by the specialty societies. However, specialty societies no longer have the final authority to approve or disapprove residency requirements. Final approval is a responsibility of the ACGME.

Each RRC reviews the programs in its specialty and recommends to the ACGME whether the program should be approved, disapproved, or put on probation. Its role is to insure that certain minimal standards are met. As an alternative to forwarding recommendations to the ACGME, RRCs may request that the authority to accredit be delegated to them. If it is, their recommendations are final.

Specialty Certification

Specialty boards separate medicine into discrete disciplines, and each board regulates the standards for its own discipline. While the boards provide the organizational structure for specialization, they do not examine whether the number of specialists being produced is appropriate or whether physicians are being appropriately trained (Stevens, 1978).

Currently, twenty-four independent specialty boards determine the educational requirements for certification in each specialty and confer certification. To be eligible for certification, a physician must: (1) meet the educational criteria of the specialty and; (2) successfully complete an accredited residency program. To become certified, the physician must pass the certification examination in that specialty. Although a licensed physician does not have to be board eligible or board certified to practice a specialty, the economic incentives are considerable. Increasingly, hospitals are requiring that their physicians be at least board eligible before they are given admitting privileges, operating room privileges, or access to specialized facilities, such as intensive care units.

chapter 5 | Biomedical Research

Biomedical research and technology development are primarily twentieth-century activities, with most of the growth occurring after World War II. In the thirty years following World War II (1945–75), expenditures for biomedical research increased dramatically, with most of the growth sponsored by the National Institutes of Health (NIH). The increased funds greatly enlarged the research function of medical schools and certain hospitals, increasing the number of residents and research fellows and significantly changing the mission of the academic health center.

The current structure and dimensions of biomedical research in academic health centers have their origins in decisions made decades ago. Policy and financing decisions made in the eighteenth, nineteenth, and early twentieth centuries established the framework for the rapid growth that occurred after World War II. A system for allocating research dollars to institutions committed to conducting research was already in place.

Background

Support for biomedical research in the eighteenth and nineteenth centuries was precarious. During the eighteenth century, autopsies were generally considered to be equivalent to grave robbing, and no respectable physician would actively pursue them (Shryock and Oki, 1951). As late as the 1860s, original research was not considered a faculty responsibility, even in the most prestigious medical schools (Ludmerer, 1985). During the 1870s and 1880s conditions began to change as a significant number of American physicians received the final years of their clinical training in Paris and Germany. Germany, the hub of medical progress, was training physicians in experimental design. However, when they returned to the United States, they found

low salaries, antiquated facilities, and little collegial support (Ludmerer, 1985). American hospitals and medical schools were generally
not receptive to scientific endeavors.

Beginning in the late 1880s, however, a critical mass of physicians
interested in biomedical research had been trained and was available
to start a new educational track. Previously, clinical medical education
was conducted as apprentice training prior to entering medical school.
In 1893, Johns Hopkins Medical School, the first school based upon
the German method of scientific inquiry, was established, and it soon
became the standard for medical education and biomedical research
in the United States. From the beginning, Johns Hopkins was a radical
departure in medical education, providing two years of instruction in
the basic sciences and two years of rigorous training in clinical sub-
jects, with students gaining experience at the hospital bedside. This
model set the stage for the development of hospitals where clinical
concepts were tested and incorporated into standard medical practice.

As physician training was moved into medical schools and as medical faculty wanted to utilize their new knowledge in clinical settings,
the hospital became an important center for biomedical research.
Johns Hopkins was distinguished from the rest of the medical schools
in 1910, because it had a state-of-the-art hospital for clinical training
and applied research (Ludmerer, 1985). In other settings, physicians
had limited opportunities for pursuing clinical research.

The Influence of Funding

Initially, most biomedical research funding came from internal
sources, usually endowment income or individual philanthropy generated by the hospital or medical school (Herdman, 1984). These small
contributions could support only limited research activities. However,
as it became apparent that biomedical research could have a positive
influence on patient care, additional funding sources became available. The success of antibiotics in treating infections during World
War I was a potent demonstration to the American public that in-
vestments in biomedical research could have significant payoffs.

Private foundations were the first major source of outside funding.
They played a critical role in the development of biomedical research
by helping to foster interactions between hospitals and medical
schools, encouraging the development of centers of excellence, and
establishing the principle of external peer review. Foundations created
by John D. Rockefeller, Cornelius Vanderbilt, Andrew Carnegie, and

J. P. Morgan began sponsoring biomedical research in the early 1900s. In Carnegie's essay, "Gospel of Wealth," health and medicine are defined as major areas of philanthropic concern. One of Carnegie's initial endeavors was to support the first laboratory for pathology in New York. In 1900, Morgan gave $1.2 million to Harvard Medical School to build a new medical school. From 1902 to 1934, approximately $154 million from philanthropic foundations went to medicine and medical education.

Foundations helped foster relationships between hospitals and medical schools. Rockefeller became involved in medicine through the affiliation of the original Rush Medical College and the University of Chicago in 1898. Later, in 1921, using the resources of the Carnegie Corporation, the Rockefeller Institute, and the Rockefeller General Education Board, a new medical center was established through the merger of Presbyterian Hospital and Columbia University's College of Physicians and Surgeons. Until this merger, most hospitals and medical schools were distinct entities without working relationships.

The second major role played by foundations was to facilitate the development of centers of excellence. Abraham Flexner, author of the 1910 Flexner Report, held that the hospital was a laboratory for clinicians. His belief that professors of clinical specialties should be salaried scientists unconstrained by the need to raise money through patient care led to the encouragement of scientific research by medical school faculty. Flexner recommended that Johns Hopkins be given $1.5 million to organize the departments of medicine, surgery, obstetrics, and pediatrics on a full-time basis. The Rockefeller Foundations also offered other medical schools, such as those at Washington University, Yale, Rochester, Vanderbilt, University of Chicago, and Harvard, funding to implement a full-time (salaried physician) system.

Implementing the full-time system in medical schools increased the research capabilities of both scientists and physicians. The graduates of these schools then brought the emphasis on science and research to other medical schools. As additional institutions followed this full-time faculty model, academic health centers developed.

As private foundations were established it became necessary to institute a process for disbursing funds. Review of research proposals by external advisory councils began in 1879, when the National Board of Health, a precursor of the NIH, made $30,000 in grants available to university scientists to study communicable disease. Private foundations established the principle of external peer review for evaluating applications. When foundations began providing substantial grants for biomedical research in the early 1900's, there was widespread distrust of the entrepreneurs who had established the foundations. Researchers and the general public were especially concerned that scientific research would be used for augmenting the personal fortunes of these individuals and not for the betterment of the general public. As a result, professional staff members at the foundations were given very limited control over awarding the grants and were not encouraged to solicit grants from individual researchers or institutions. The primary role of the foundation was to select outside reviewers for grant proposals and to manage the disbursement of funds.

The Initial Federal Role

Federal involvement in biomedical research began slowly, limited initially to public health activities (Lierman, 1983). The Public Health Service opened a small hygienic laboratory in 1887 at the Merchant Marine Hospital on Staten Island, New York, which conducted intramural research on immunology (Fredrickson, 1981). As the number and size of academic medical centers began to grow and the benefits of medical research became apparent, the existing sources of support for biomedical research, internal funds, and private foundations, became insufficient. During the 1920s, private foundations began to encourage federal involvement in biomedical research. In congressional testimony, George Vincent, president of the Rockefeller Foundations, argued that, despite progress in our knowledge of disease through laboratory investigation, the federal government had a duty to participate in and support these efforts and that the United States should follow the lead of England and Germany, which were already officially supporting scientific research. He also argued that the federal government should give the researchers flexibility to develop their own research projects (Fosdick, 1962).

In the 1920s the administration and the Congress debated the appropriate federal government role in biomedical research, and numerous compromises reached during congressional debates influenced the future direction of federal involvement in biomedical research (Harden, 1986). One major debate concerned the level of funding. The Budget Office wanted to keep the program as small as possible and to limit the extent of extramural programs, while proponents of federal funding for research argued for a major financial commitment that would encourage extramural research.

A second debate focused on the role of the federal government in relation to the private sector. Many federal policymakers believed that the private sector should be the primary funding source for biomedical research, with the federal government providing only selective, limited support. Leaders in the private sector argued for broad-based federal support.

In 1930, the Ransdell Act established the National Institutes of Health and authorized $750,000 for the construction of two buildings and the creation of a system of fellowships. In 1937, Congress authorized the National Cancer Institute. However, prior to World War II, the National Institutes of Health was not a major supporter of medical research. In 1940, NIH had a budget of $707,000, of which only $277,000 went to research grants. In the same year, private foundations gave $4,700,000 for research grants, almost seven times the entire NIH budget (Strickland, 1972).

During World War II, federal spending on biomedical research increased substantially. Military leaders recognized that preventing the spread of disease and treating soldiers quickly was important to the war effort. As a result, the military developed a major program, the Committee on Medical Research (CMR), which provided funding to universities. The CMR was directed to mobilize the nation's medical and scientific personnel and to recommend support for areas of biomedical research being conducted by universities, hospitals, and other scientific agencies. All of the resources were spent on extramural research, since the military had minimal biomedical research facilities. The committee distributed $15 million to 450 universities and employed 5,500 scientists. From the beginning, funding decisions were left to panels of independent scientists, and the government played a laissez-faire role during the life of the project (Stevens, 1978).

In 1944, Congress passed the Public Health Service Act, which gave NIH the legislative basis to give grants and fellowships in a manner similar to the Committee on Medical Research. When the war was over, the infrastructure for the federal support of biomedical research was firmly established, and the responsibility for monitoring the remaining university-based research projects administered by the CMR was transferred to the National Institutes of Health. In November 1945, President Harry Truman's health message included the expansion of federally supported biomedical research as one of his four major programs. After World War II, expenditures on biomedical research increased dramatically.

Table 5-1. Financing Sources for Biomedical Research, 1960–1987 (percent)

Year	Federal	State and Local	Private Sector
1960	50.5	5.1	44.2
1965	62.1	4.7	33.1
1970	58.5	5.9	35.4
1975	60.2	6.0	33.6
1980	59.3	6.3	34.4
1985	50.9	6.5	42.6
1986	47.2	6.9	45.8
1987	47.2	6.6	46.1

Source: Based on data from U.S. Department of Health and Human Services, 1987.

Federal Funding

Sources of financing biomedical research between 1960 and 1985 are presented in table 5-1. The federal government supports between 50 and 60 percent; state and local governments fund only a small proportion. The private sector, both corporation and philanthropic donors, provides the remaining thirty to forty percent via internally and externally sponsored research activities.

Federal funding for biomedical research is distributed through NIH, the Public Health Service (PHS), the Veterans' Administration (VA) system, the National Science Foundation (NSF), and other agencies. The single largest source of federal support is the NIH, which consistently accounts for more than two-thirds of total federal funds.

NIH's expenditures on research grants increased from $142,000 in 1945 to $4 million in 1947, when most of the Committee on Medical Research contracts were transferred to the NIH. They have grown substantially each year since then.

The distribution of NIH appropriations from 1940 to 1985 is displayed in table 5-2. The federal government provided limited funds for extramural research during the early years. Beginning in the mid-1950s, government allocations increased, and NIH became a major influence in the development of biomedical research both on its own campus through intramural funding and in academic health centers across the country via extramural grants. Although appropriations have grown significantly in current dollars, in constant dollars, NIH's purchasing power for research and training grants peaked during the late 1960s (figure 5-1). Since the early seventies, there have been

Table 5-2.   Appropriations by the National Institutes of Health, 1940–1985 (thousands of current dollars)

Year	Extramural Research Grants	Internal Operations	Total
1940	277	430	707
1945	142	2,693	2,835
1950	36,754	15,392	52,146
1955	54,331	25,937	81,268
1960	334,430	95,570	430,000
1965	875,199	183,793	1,058,992
1970	1,210,320	313,020	1,523,340
1975	1,386,280	703,615	2,089,897
1980	2,356,062	1,069,623	3,425,685
1985	3,772,327	1,349,230	5,121,557

Source: U.S. Department of Health and Human Services, 1984; and unpublished data from the National Institutes of Health.

small incremental increases in constant dollars for research grants. Due to a perceived surplus of physicians, training and fellowship grants, however, have fallen off steadily since the late 1960s.

Private Industry Funding

There is little information on private industry involvement in funding medical research and development. A recent survey of biotechnology firms suggests that their level of involvement in biomedical research is increasing (Blumenthal, Gluck, and Louis, 1986a). The survey indicates that 46 percent of all firms in the biotechnology industry support research in academic health centers. Furthermore, 31 percent of the firms that support university--based research invest more than 10 percent of their research and development budgets on university campuses. Industry provided 16 to 24 percent of all funds for biomedical research available to academic health centers in 1984 (Blumenthal, Gluck, and Louis, 1986a).

Pharmaceutical firms and equipment manufacturers conducting clinical trials in the United States provide support. In addition to funding the cost of the drug or equipment, corporations theoretically fund tests or days of care beyond the standard medical procedures necessitated by the clinical trial.

In many foreign countries, most of the cost of the clinical trial is paid for indirectly by the government through national health insur-

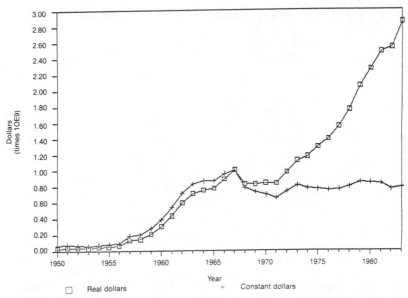

Figure 5-1.   Biomedical Research Grants from the National Institutes of Health, 1950–1983

ance. This creates an economic incentive for U.S. manufacturers to conduct clinical trials outside the United States, where hospital-based drug trials cost considerably less and can be conducted more quickly. Consequently, some pharmaceutical companies are setting up bases of operation in European countries for this reason. In the past, many of the trials had to be repeated in the United States to receive Food and Drug Administration (FDA) approval, because other countries' policies are generally not as stringent as those of the United States. Recently, however, the FDA has become increasingly willing to accept clinical trials conducted in foreign countries as long as they meet specified regulations. Following the change, pharmaceutical companies and biotechnological equipment manufacturers increased their use of foreign sites for final testing of their products. To the extent that clinical drug trials are increasingly conducted outside of the United States, funds flowing to teaching hospitals to conduct these studies will necessarily diminish.

The Distribution of Biomedical Research

Currently, most biomedical research is concentrated in a very few academic centers, with 75 percent of NIH funds going to forty institutions and 44 percent going to only twenty institutions. This concentration may place a significant financial burden on the hospitals serving as clinical sites for research, or it may provide them with a marketing edge, since they are known to have state-of-the-art technology and clinicians. It also raises public policy concerns about relying on a small number of institutions for the majority of our nation's biomedical research.

For years, there have been debates among academics and policymakers relating to the desirability of the extreme concentration of research funding in relatively few institutions of higher education (Perry, Challoner, and Oberst, 1981; Arnow, 1983). The argument supporting this concentration says that biomedical science on the cutting edge of a discipline requires the use of large multidisciplinary teams of investigators. Universities that receive substantial grant support may have the widest variety and highest quality of research activity. This in turn attracts new, highly skilled, successful scientists, which again increases the possibility that research funding will flow to that university. Table 5-3 displays the top twenty recipients of NIH research grants in 1985. The total funds awarded to these institutions, nearly $1.2 billion, represents 44 percent of all external funds available through NIH.

This funding for basic science and clinical research includes all money awarded to the university, not just the teaching hospital. In fact, these funds seldom go directly to teaching hospitals but instead to the medical school. Data on the extent of research conducted in teaching hospitals is difficult to obtain. The commonly held belief is that university-affiliated teaching hospitals are very involved in clinical research, but there is no data to support this.

A second distributional issue involves the recipient of funding. NIH awards research grants primarily to the individual, not the institution. This policy allows NIH to concentrate evaluation on the quality of the proposal and the promise of the individual(s) involved. In 1985, nine percent of the annual funds from NIH were, however, earmarked for clinical research centers distributed across the country. These centers received an annual grant to support general research conducted at the hospital.

The Cost of Biomedical Research

Unlike clinical education, where the cost has been analyzed in a variety of studies, very little is known about the cost of biomedical re-

Table 5-3.   Top Twenty Recipients of NIH Research Grant Support, 1985

Institution	NIH Support (dollars)
The Johns Hopkins University	89,095,000
University of California, Berkeley	81,280,000
Columbia University	71,502,000
Yale University	71,441,000
Stanford University	71,030,000
University of Washington	70,886,000
University of Pennsylvania	68,956,000
Harvard University	68,916,000
University of California, Los Angeles	64,754,000
University of Minnesota	56,041,000
Washington University	55,346,000
University of Wisconsin, Madison	54,111,000
Yeshiva University	51,543,000
University of Michigan	50,352,000
University of California, San Diego	49,812,000
Duke University	47,751,000
Cornell University	43,070,000
University of Chicago	42,900,000
Massachusetts Institute of Technology	41,330,000
University of New York Medical Center	40,456,000

Source: Based on data from U.S. Department of Health and Human Services, 1985.
Note: Includes all NIH funds to the university; most funds go to the university's medical school.

search to the hospital (Aaron, 1986; Peterson, 1986). Most hospital administrators show little concern about the costs associated with conducting research, and therefore it has yet to become a major issue. This is not especially surprising, given that a substantial proportion of all biomedical research occurs in a limited number of clinical settings.

The Medicare prospective payment system, however, is beginning to make this issue more visible (Davis, 1985). According to the Prospective Payment Assessment Commission (ProPAC, 1987) "third-party cost-reimbursement structure concealed a significant amount of subsidization for the patient care component of clinical research. This occurred because the cost of caring for patients being treated with new therapies and treatments is frequently higher than the cost of research from patient care. Furthermore, it is frequently not possible to separate the costs of research from patient care" p. 69 (ProPAC).

Many of the costs associated with research are incorporated into the hospital's cost base. Since the majority of the hospital's revenue comes from patient care, hospital-based research is funded primarily through patient revenues via cross-subsidies. Generally, biomedical research can be split into two major categories—sponsored and unsponsored projects, both of which may increase hospital costs.

Sponsored Research

Sponsored research involves clinical and basic science projects explicitly funded either by public or private sources or by the hospital, using internally generated funds. With sponsored research, the investigator is expected to determine the direct costs associated with the research and submit these costs to the funding agency as part of the application. Sponsors generally pay direct costs, including wages and fringe benefits, materials, supplies, travel, any additional laboratory tests or days of hospital care that may occur as the result of the research protocol, and other expenses associated with conducting the research. External sponsors also fund overhead costs (which they call indirect costs), including expenses such as administration, plant maintenance, depreciation and interest on buildings and equipment, utilities, compliance with federal regulations, and other overhead expenses associated with the research. Normal patient care costs are not funded through the grants.

Although sponsored projects are theoretically funded to cover all of the research costs, it is unclear whether or not they pay the full costs. Some biomedical research may be sponsored but underfunded. For example, in the clinical trial of a new drug, the cost of the drug is likely to be covered under supplies. However, in the event that the standard course of treatment is altered, additional tests or procedures may be required to treat the patient. Researchers may not be able to identify all of the additional services that may be necessary, a priori. In addition, since total cost is a factor in the evaluation of a research project, there is an incentive to underestimate project costs to reduce the total cost of the project. As a result, unanticipated costs will be absorbed by the hospital or third-party payors, filed as a supplemental request for funds to the funding agency, or passed on to the patient.

The hospital also incurs costs when it supports research projects through internal funds. The cost of using a new piece of equipment is usually greater than the cost after the technology has diffused, because the cost has by then been lowered and the medical standard of practice established (Anderson and Steinberg, 1984a). These research projects add to the hospital's costs with little or no immediate offsetting revenue, but they may have long-run payoffs as the hospital becomes known for having the latest technology. The cost of internally funded projects is generally unknown. As a point of reference, Johns Hopkins Hospital spends approximately 3 to 4 percent of its annual operating budget on internally sponsored projects.

Unsponsored Research

Unsponsored research involves all of the research conducted in the hospital that is not explicitly funded by internal or external sources. This can involve surgeons using the operating room an additional fifteen minutes to develop or perfect a new surgical technique; radiologists requesting both an MRI (magnetic resonance imaging) and a CT (computerized tomography) scan for a patient because the physician is unsure of the relative strengths and weakness of each technology in a specific instance; or clinical case studies that might require review and evaluation of all patients with a specific illness treated in that institution during a given period of time. Unsponsored research frequently occurs when new products or procedures are developed and clinicians are unsure whether the old standard or the new is the most efficacious (Anderson and Steinberg, 1984a). The cost of unsponsored research is difficult to analyze, since the magnitude of such research conducted in academic health centers is generally unknown. Some of this research may appear to be fairly low cost, such as clinical case studies requiring a retrospective review of patient charts over a specified period of time. Others may be more expensive, such as those involving operating room time or additional ancillary tests.

The cost of unsponsored research has been largely unquestioned by the institutions supporting it. Although the leaders of major academic health centers whom we interviewed speculated that the cost could be very large, they have been largely unconcerned with the extent to which these activities contribute to the higher cost of producing patient care. These administrators also appear to be unwilling to significantly control the hospitals' involvement in unsponsored research. Major academic health centers sponsor biomedical research as part of their mission and have generally accepted the unreimbursed costs of research as a cost of that mission.

To date, no comprehensive, quantitative studies have examined how the cost of biomedical research contributes to the cost of running a hospital. The National Center for Health Services Research in conjunction with the National Cancer Institute is conducting a study on the cost differences between cancer patients in an experimental research protocol versus patients with comparable diagnoses receiving conventional treatment. It will be difficult to generalize from this study, because it focuses on one type of patient; and the results may be biased, since most protocol patients do not have complications or comorbid conditions.

A second study, conducted by the Commonwealth Task Force on Academic Health Centers, has been developed to identify the scope of underfunded and unsponsored research conducted at five major teaching hospitals and to quantify the cost of this activity to the hospital. Results indicate that 20 to 32 percent of the costs associated with caring for patients involved in research protocols were covered by the hospital. These expenses were concentrated in five categories; bed days, laboratory testing, radiology, medical/surgical supplies, and clinic visits. The study also revealed that the cost to the hospital varied by source of funding. Private industry-sponsored research paid for a larger share of total costs than government-sponsored projects. Because of the limited scope of this study, it is not possible to make generalizations relevant to the universe of academic health centers. However, these results do suggest that hospitals sponsor a portion of the cost of research.

The analysis presented in chapter 1 uses research fellows as a proxy for the extent of underfunded research conducted in the hospital. The results suggest that each research fellow adds twenty-three dollars to the operating cost per discharge after the direct costs associated with the research are removed from the cost comparison. While research fellows are a crude proxy for the scope of research activity, it does suggest that research may add to the total cost of the hospital.

The Financing of Biomedical Research

Earlier in this chapter, we discussed the development of financing for biomedical research and looked at trends in the sources and level of funding. In this section, the role of the teaching hospital in financing biomedical research and technology development is reviewed.

Understanding the financing of biomedical research is complicated because of the intricate relationships between the entities involved. Generally, a research grant is awarded to the medical school, which may then allocate resources to the hospital on a project-specific basis to cover direct costs of the project. Many times, however, resources are bartered between the medical school and the hospital, so that funds are not actually exchanged. Thus it is difficult to determine if adequate funds have been transferred to the hospital to cover the costs of clinical research, since the costs of conducting the research may be unknown.

In addition to direct costs funded through the grant, there may be unfunded direct costs, if the project is underfunded. Investigators are expected to identify all direct costs in advance. However, because research applications are judged, in part, on direct cost, there are incentives to minimize cost by underestimating, for instance, tests required or additional days in the hospital. Unless there is a mechanism in place to compare actual costs with projected costs, the difference may be absorbed by the hospital and implicitly funded via patient care revenues.

Academic medical centers also fund biomedical research using faculty salary support. Most commonly, they provide partial funding for young physicians to reduce clinical responsibilities, thus freeing time and encouraging faculty to pursue research interests. Funds for salary support may originate from a variety of sources, including general operating funds, discretionary funds at the department level, or faculty practice plans (chapter 2).

Hospitals often explicitly sponsor research, typically funding technology development and clinical research by sponsoring new programs within the institution. Medical technology develops in stages, moving from basic research, to laboratory production and testing, to refinement via clinical application before it is broadly disseminated and incorporated into standard medical practice. Academic hospitals frequently become engaged during the refinement stage when the technology is still considered experimental. Examples include development of clinical applications for the MRI. Sponsored MRI programs fund further experimentation and the development of clinical uses of the technology. At this stage, physicians use both MRI and the currently accepted medical standard, CT scanning, or another radiologic technique. Results from these tests are compared, and physicians determine appropriate uses of the new technology, for example whether MRI should be a substitute for or a complement to the other technology. Eventually, appropriate clinical uses of MRI are established, and where there was once repetition in testing, the new technology will likely take over as the new standard (Anderson and Steinberg, 1984a).

Another example is the development of new surgical procedures. Transplant programs have been developed in numerous academic hospitals. An institution's commitment to a program of this type requires funding for additional support staff, space, specialized facilities, state-of-the-art equipment, and sometimes additional physicians. In the early stages of development, these programs are very expensive, because fixed costs are high and volume is low.

Funds for hospital-sponsored projects may come from a variety of sources, depending on the organizational structure of the institution. Historically, revenues from patient care services were used to support some of the research activities in major academic health centers (Kahn, 1984). In institutions where faculty practice plans have been created, the plans may be taxed to establish a discretionary account for the hospital or the medical school dean (MacLeod, Rockette, and Schwarz, 1987). In some institutions, university research foundations have been created to generate income by patenting and marketing research ideas that have commercial applications (Omenn, 1982; Bloomberg, Marylander, and Yeager, 1987). These foundations provide arrangements that retain key faculty members and create incentives to emphasize clinical service. They generally provide supplemental income to the individual faculty member; negotiate a balance among practice, teaching, and research; and generate unrestricted funds for the institution. Funds generated through this mechanism can be retained or redistributed by the institution within the academic community to support new research. To the extent that these funds are used to fund research that is underfunded or that is financed via internal funds, the hospital receives spillover benefits.

The Control of Biomedical Research Funds

A new issue for teaching hospitals is the financial control of research grants. Generally, funds for research grants are awarded to the medical school, and the hospital may or may not fully recover the direct costs related to activities conducted in the hospital. As a consequence, increasing attention is being given to the costs of research.

In addition to direct costs, sponsors also fund overhead costs. But overhead cost rates vary dramatically across institutions (Kutina, Bruss, and Paich, 1985). At the top twenty institutions receiving NIH funds, overhead costs ranged from a low of 21.42 percent at the University of California at San Francisco, to a high of 44.37 percent at Yeshiva University. Traditionally, payments for overhead costs have been retained by the university or medical school. Hospitals rarely receive a share of the overhead reimbursement for indirect costs associated with these projects. However, this practice may be changing, and hospitals are beginning to argue for a share of the overhead.

The growing involvement of private industry in biomedical research has caused some observers to believe that its involvement lessens the control the faculty investigator has over the research agenda. Relman (1985) has suggested that "entrepreneurialism among physicians is a widespread and rapidly growing phenomenon, which is creating conflicts of interest in almost all sectors of the medical profession" (p. 730). When investigators who report new research developments with commercial application own equity or have other kinds of financial interest in a company whose fortunes are affected by the result, conflicts of interest may develop.

Critics of the privatization of biomedical research are concerned that it will change the nature of research conducted at universities. Results from such research have traditionally been treated as public goods, that is, the results were disseminated quickly and were not considered proprietary. In the private sector, research results are frequently treated as trade secrets and cannot be published or freely discussed with colleagues or students (Blumenthal, Gluck, and Louis, 1986b). This could impede the "free, rapid and unbiased dissemination of research results." Blumenthal, Gluck, and Louis (1986b) revealed that 24 percent of the university faculty supported by industrial grants were constrained by agreements made with the corporate sponsor, such that the research results were the property of the sponsor and could not be published without their consent.

Summary

In summary, while biomedical research is not currently a major issue, there is much potential for controversy. Biomedical research is an expensive proposition and is not completely financed by those sponsoring the research. Further, there is concern about who is controlling the research and where it is being conducted. This suggests that biomedical research and technology development will soon become a major topic of public policy interest.

chapter 6 | Uncompensated Care

In 1986, an estimated thirty-seven million people were without health insurance in the United States some time during the year, and an additional 20–30 million were underinsured. The problems of the uninsured, the underinsured, and uncompensated hospital care are beginning to attract considerable attention for several reasons.

First, the number of people without insurance for some part of the year is growing. As shown in table 6-1, the number of uninsured persons under age sixty-five on any given day increased from 26 million in 1978 to almost 37 million in 1986. In 1986, more than 17 percent of the population under age sixty-five was uninsured at some time during the year. This increase has been attributed partially to changes in eligibility criteria for public programs and to changes in the structure of American industry.

Second, a number of empirical studies demonstrate a relationship between health coverage, use of health services, and health outcomes. The rate of hospitalization, the average length of stay, and the use of physician services are all lower for the uninsured than for the insured populations. Of greater concern is that lack of health coverage appears to be associated with increases in morbidity and mortality.

Third, although most hospitals provide services to people who cannot pay their bills, the cost of providing uncompensated care is spread unevenly across hospitals and insurers. Some hospitals, because of ownership, geographic location, or charitable commitment, admit a much higher proportion of nonpaying or underpaying patients than others. Some third-party payors, in particular the commercial insurance companies, report that hospitals increase the rates for private paying patients, forcing the charge-based payors to absorb a disproportionate share of uncompensated care costs.

Fourth, state and local governments are more concerned about the burden of charity care. State and local governments typically support public hospitals. With the rising demand for services in public

Table 6-1. The Nonaged Uninsured, 1978–1986

Year	Number of Uninsured (millions)	Uninsured as Percentage of Population under Sixty-five
1978	26.0	13.6
1980	28.6	14.6
1982	30.7	15.2
1984	35.1	17.1
1986	36.9	17.6

Source: Adapted from Sulvetta and Swartz, 1986; for 1986 estimate, personal communication with Swartz, August 1988.

hospitals, hospital care is consuming a greater share of state and local budgets. Ultimately, taxpayers subsidize hospital expenses for patients without adequate health insurance coverage.

Finally, it is becoming more difficult for hospitals to finance the cost of caring for the uninsured. In the past, hospitals relied upon funds raised through philanthropy, public appropriations, and patient revenues to subsidize the cost of treating poor and uninsured patients. However, philanthropic contributions are decreasing as a percentage of total health expenditures (Stevens, 1982). At the same time, price competition is restricting the ability of hospitals to raise prices to paying patients in order to cover the costs of those who cannot pay in full. Consequently, some hospitals are taking actions to make it more difficult for uninsured people to receive medical attention. These actions exacerbate the difficulties that already face the uninsured who seek hospital care, as well as the financial burden on those hospitals that continue to admit them.

The confluence of these factors—the growing number of uninsured and underinsured persons; the vulnerability of people without insurance; the unequal distribution of uncompensated care costs across hospitals and payors; the relative burden on state and local governments and ultimately on taxpayers; and the diminishing ability of hospitals to cover uncompensated costs through cross-subsidies—has once again drawn public attention to the issues of how we provide and pay for health services for the poor.

Background

Historical Issues

Issues concerning care for the poor are not new to the United States. Debate over local responsibility for the poor dates back to the settlement of the colonies. Drawing directly on English precedent and the role of the church, early American settlers arrived in this country believing that communities should assume some obligation to provide for those who were unable to care for themselves. The American settlers, like their English counterparts, believed that the method of caring for the poor should be controlled at the local level. Families were encouraged to take care of their own; but most communities assumed responsibility for the poor, destitute, insane, and aged who had no other source of care.

The level of community support, however, has been extremely variable. One of the most important determinants of the level of support was the concept of the deserving poor. In the late seventeenth century, there was a proliferation of almshouses established to offer the "deserving poor" an opportunity to support themselves in the community. To some extent, almshouses were considered agents of social reform; the poor, it was believed, could become productive members of the community if given food, shelter, and some religious training (Katz, 1984). A related argument was that health and other services should be made available in the spirit of "enlightened capitalism"; that is, the belief that the infusion of health and other social services would keep the work force healthy and productive (Rosner, 1982).

By the mid-nineteenth century, most counties had established their own almshouse, and in many states, mental asylums were established to house persons considered to be insane or otherwise threatening to the community's well-being. Some communities created pest houses to isolate persons with highly infectious diseases. Toward the end of the nineteenth century, however, few individuals continued to believe in the social value of the almshouse, for they had become shelters for social misfits and were not effective in promoting industry or intemperance among the deserving poor (Katz, 1984). By the late nineteenth century, therefore, the nature of community support for the poor had been transformed dramatically. No longer linked with a belief in productive outcomes, the more expansive periods of support for the poor were coincident with a perceived threat to the health and safety of the general community (Rosner, 1982).

Public Support

Hospitals were founded approximately a hundred years after the establishment of the first almshouses. The first hospital, the Pennsylvania Hospital, was established in 1751, with the help of Benjamin Franklin. Many others were built during the next hundred years. Most early hospitals were private institutions financed through a combination of public and private funds.

As cities became more densely populated, the first government hospitals were set up to control the spread of infectious diseases, such as cholera and diarrhea. Although both state and local governments continued to support private institutions, they also built their own hospitals. Federal government support for general hospitals was very limited, although as early as 1798, the first Merchant Marine hospital was established.

During the early decades of the nineteenth century, public financial support for voluntary hospitals became fairly commonplace. State governments made payments to hospitals to help cover the expense of caring for the poor (Stevens, 1974). For example, in 1816 Massachusetts began making annual grants to the Eye and Ear Infirmary and to the New England Hospital for Women and Children. States and municipal governments provided grants to specific hospitals with a large share of charity cases. In cities with large numbers of immigrants, voluntary hospitals received government payments to relieve the burden on government hospitals in the area. Where there were no government hospitals, state governments paid voluntary hospitals for providing care to the poor.

Public support for hospital care was substantial by the turn of the twentieth century. A 1903 survey of 1,493 general and special U.S. hospitals (including 220 government hospitals, 831 private hospitals, and 442 ecclesiastical hospitals) found that hospitals had received $8.5 million from public sources. Of this, $2.3 million were allocated to private hospitals, while $6.2 million were allocated to public hospitals. Government support amounted to 29.9 percent of total hospital revenues. The level of public support for private hospitals varied significantly from state to state (Stevens, 1974).

While it is not clear that all government funds were appropriated to care for the poor, it is generally agreed that public support was contingent upon the level of charity care provided by the hospital. In fact, until the 1920s the distinction between public and voluntary hospitals was often blurred, because both received substantial public funds and both were expected to provide a substantial amount of charity care (Starr, 1982).

The Hospital's Role in the Twentieth Century

By the beginning of the twentieth century, U.S. hospitals began to assume more of the characteristics associated with the modern hospital. This was a time of substantial improvements in the training of medical professionals and in the levels of facilities, equipment, and hygiene. As a result of these technical advances, nonpoor individuals, who earlier would have been treated in their home by private physicians, chose to receive medical care in a hospital setting. The demand for hospital services grew rapidly and, as a result, the hospital sector expanded markedly. Between 1873 and 1927, the number of hospitals increased from 170 to over 4,000 (Rosner, 1982).

The poor continued to be treated in public, voluntary, and religious-sponsored institutions. Voluntary hospitals, although increasingly interested in serving private, paying patients, continued to provide care for the poor both to fulfill their charitable missions and to facilitate clinical education. Municipal and county hospitals tended to serve primarily poor patients with highly infectious diseases or those with chronic illnesses associated with venereal disease, mental illness, and old age. Religious and ethnic hospitals, funded mostly by their endowments, tended to serve their respective constituencies. Almshouses and mental asylums were still available to treat the "undesirable" poor.

Concomitant with the increasing demand for hospital services by private paying patients was an apparent shift in public attitudes toward care for the poor. As American cities became more densely populated, large pockets of poverty were created, which served to focus attention on the association between poverty and bad health. Xenophobia, triggered by the infusion of large numbers of immigrants, contributed to the declining commitment to care for the poor (Higham, 1975). Whereas earlier it was believed that the poor could and should be transformed into productive members of the work force, by the late nineteenth century, the commitment to the poor appeared ambivalent at best, perhaps based on the assumption that the poor were responsible for their own lack of economic success—and bad health (Katz, 1984). Community leaders had a choice: they could in a sense, blame the poor for their condition and bad health by cutting back on charity care; or they could find some way to provide health services. Ultimately, the community recognized an interest in providing services to the poor even if only to control the spread of disease.

As the quality of hospital care improved, the demand from private patients for hospital services increased. Voluntary hospitals began to limit services to the poor (Rosner, 1982). Concerned about the high costs of charity care, hospitals of the late nineteenth century established three mechanisms to limit their potential financial liability.

They could (1) reduce the amount of free care provided; (2) increase the number of private paying patients; or (3) eliminate unnecessary use of hospital services (Rosner, 1982). These policies are still being pursued by some hospitals today.

Some communities debated whether private hospitals should continue to provide charity services or whether, instead, the burden of charity care should be shifted to public hospitals. To illustrate the sensitivity of hospital planners and administrators to problems associated with charity care, a 1904 survey of administrators of major New York hospitals asked whether they believed that hospitals should be divided into two groups. In one group would be hospitals with patients who could pay for their treatment, in the other would be hospitals with only charity patients. The administrators rejected the idea of two classes of hospitals. Administrators of the voluntary hospitals were concerned about losing charitable donations if all poor patients were treated in municipal hospitals (Starr, 1982).

The Government's Role in the Twentieth Century

Public programs entitling individuals to health care did not exist in the United States before the twentieth century. However, in 1908, the U.S. government followed the lead of several European countries by establishing worker's compensation programs to cover the hospital expenses of federal civilian employees who were injured at work. Shortly thereafter, most state governments established similar programs for state employees. At that time, neither federal nor state governments were prepared to go the additional step taken by most European countries of adopting a national health program to assure access to all.

Since the early decades of the twentieth century, U.S. policy makers have considered the idea of national health insurance. The first president to push the idea of national health insurance was Theodore Roosevelt, who argued that no country could be strong whose people are sick and poor. In the late 1920s the question of entitling individuals to health coverage was among the issues considered by the Committee on the Costs of Medical Care. This privately funded independent body composed of economists, physicians, and public health specialists was formed to address concerns about the costs and distribution of medical services. In their final report, published in 1933, the committee emphasized the need to reduce economic barriers to medical care through the expansion of voluntary health insurance plans. It opposed compulsory health insurance on two grounds: first, such insurance would represent an "unprecedented" subsidy from government; second, it would freeze existing problems into place. Eight of the thirty-five signatories of the final report dissented from the majority opinion on compulsory health insurance; they argued that voluntary plans would not help the poor, who most needed protection against the high costs of medical care (Starr, 1982).

During the 1920s and 1930s, the American Associates for Labor Legislation lobbied for national health insurance. They advanced three basic arguments for extending medical insurance beyond workman's compensation: first, individuals should have insurance to cover the costs borne by hospitals for an illness or accident; second, poverty in the country would diminish, because insurance redistributes income; and third, insurance reduces the long-term costs of illness by financing better medical care when it is needed. The Social Security Act, passed by the Congress in 1935, included disability insurance, workman's compensation, and a pension benefit, but not health insurance.

During the 1930s, Blue Cross plans were established. Designed in part to assure the financial stability of hospitals, Blue Cross insured individuals for the costs of hospital services. By 1940, as many as six million Americans, nearly 4.5 percent of the population, were enrolled. Meanwhile, Congress continued to consider ways to broaden health coverage for the poor. The Wagner-Murray-Dingell bill, for example, was introduced to entitle the "very needy" to health services. Senator Robert Taft articulated the views of the bill's opponents: any government-sponsored health care was an "aberrant necessity rather than being generally desirable," and eligibility for benefits should be discretionary rather than a right (Stevens, 1982). The legislation was defeated. As the number of people with private health insurance increased, interest in public health insurance waned, as many believed that government involvement would be duplicative of private efforts.

Early Federal Programs   The first direct congressional response to the problems of the poor and uninsured was the creation of a program to provide funds to hospitals that offered charity care. The Hospital Survey and Construction Act (Hill-Burton act), passed in 1946, was designed explicitly to encourage care for the poor by restricting federal funds for hospital construction to hospitals that agreed to provide care to the poor. The Congress in effect recognized an obligation to the poor without directly entitling them to medical services (Blumstein, 1986). This was important legislation, because the focus of federal debate turned from expanding coverage for the poor to providing resources to hospitals that treated the poor.

Later laws passed by Congress enabled the federal government to share the cost of services to welfare recipients. Under the original Social Security Act, federal funds could be used only to support the administrative costs of the welfare programs and to share in the cost of cash grants to individuals. Some states chose instead to implement programs that paid providers directly for rendering services to welfare recipients. In 1950, the Social Security Act was amended, allowing the federal government to share the cost of vendor payments. Congress enacted the Medical Assistance Program for the Aged (MAA) in 1960, which established a federal-state program to pay providers for health care services delivered to individuals whose income was above the state's old age assistance levels. Federal laws governing vendor payment programs were not very restrictive; states could implement vendor payment programs for any or all categorical assistance programs (including MAA) and could cover different services under each program. In 1964 vendor payments to hospitals amounted to $480 million, or 5.75 percent of total hospital expenses (Lave, 1967).

Medicare and Medicaid   In 1965, the Medicare and Medicaid programs were established. Medicare consists of two separate but complementary programs: hospital insurance for hospital, skilled nursing facility, and home health services; and supplementary medical insurance for the services of physicians, outpatient medical services, and the costs of durable medical equipment and prostheses. The Medicare program had three primary objectives: (1) to protect the elderly from the financial hardship resulting from large medical expenses; (2) to improve access to the health care system; and (3) to eliminate the differences in the use of health care services between the poor and the nonpoor elderly. Currently, over 95 percent of the aged population are enrolled in both Medicare programs.

A major initial concern in Congress was that hospitals and other providers would not participate in the program. To gain the cooperation of providers, Congress incorporated into the Medicare program many of the standard features of the Blue Cross/Blue Shield plans. The most important features included giving beneficiaries the freedom to choose their own providers, cost-based reimbursement for institutional providers, and fee-for-service reimbursement for physicians. By explicit design, Medicare reimbursement rates excluded costs associated with either bad debt or charity care for non-Medicare beneficiaries. This policy remains in effect today.

The success of the program in providing health services to poor elderly people can be measured using indicators of utilization. Before the Medicare program was enacted, utilization of health services was inversely related to family income (Rice, 1964). In fact, the observed difference in hospital use by insurance status (which was highly related to income) was one of the important factors giving impetus to the enactment of the program. In 1969, utilization of hospital services by Medicare recipients was still strongly influenced by income and race (Davis and Reynolds, 1975). By the mid-1970s, many of these differences had disappeared (Ruther and Dobson, 1981; Link, Long, and Settle, 1982). While not all of the change in relative hospital utilization can be attributed to the success of the public programs, surely some of it can be.

The Medicaid program, in contrast to Medicare, was designed specifically to cover the cost of providing hospital and other medical services to specified groups of low-income Americans. Medicaid is administered by the states, subject to federal guidelines. The federal government establishes broad program requirements and allows the states to determine specific eligibility, benefit, and reimbursement policies. The states are required to cover all persons receiving cash assistance under the Supplemental Security Income program and Aid to Families with Dependent Children program. States have the option of covering the medically needy populations (i.e., aged, blind, disabled, and single-parent families whose income is above the cash assistance level but is considered too low to pay for medical expenses), of establishing spend-down programs (to pay the medical expenses of people whose medical expenses bring their income below the state-determined Medicaid eligibility level), and of covering families with unemployed fathers. The Medicaid program thus perpetuates both the practice of making care for the poor essentially a local—in this case state—responsibility and the concept of the deserving poor.

Each state is required to provide a basic benefit package to all eligible beneficiaries. Federally mandated benefits include both inpatient and outpatient hospital services, physician services, laboratory and X-ray services, screening and diagnostic services for children, and home care and nursing home care for adults. States may elect to provide other services and to receive a federal match for them.

Medicaid is not a comprehensive health care program for the poor. The number of poor persons covered by Medicaid is largely a function of income levels and other criteria used to establish eligibility for the cash assistance programs. The proportion of the poor and near poor covered by Medicaid increased from 32 percent in 1969 to 63 percent in 1975, but steadily decreased thereafter. By 1985, only 46 percent of the poor and near poor were covered by Medicaid (U.S. Senate, 1985).

The Medicaid program originally required that hospitals be paid on the same basis as Medicare (cost-based reimbursement) and that Medicaid recipients have freedom of choice among providers. Both of these restrictions were eliminated in 1981, and states were given more flexibility to design their own reimbursement and service delivery systems.

To date, the Medicaid program represents the most significant federal and state commitment to providing the poor access to health care. Between 1964 and 1981, hospital utilization by the poor increased from 138 to 202 discharged per 1,000, while those of nonpoor Americans increased slightly, from 126 to 131 discharges per 1,000 (Blendon, 1986). Medicaid coverage resulted directly in increased service utilization by the poor: utilization rates by the poor covered by Medicaid were three times higher than those of the poor who were uninsured (Wilensky and Berk, 1982).

It is difficult to determine the direct impact of the Medicaid program on the health status of poor Americans. Since 1965, significant improvements have occurred in medical practice and medical technology, and these improvements may confound the influence of the Medicaid program. Nonetheless, proxies for health status of low-income persons suggest that substantial improvements have occurred following the implementation of the Medicaid program. Infant death rates for nonwhite children have dropped by more than 40 percent since 1965 (National Center for Health Statistics, 1985). Deaths from diseases for which medical care can be life saving have also decreased (Rogers, Blendon, and Maloney, 1982). The Medicaid program appears to be responsible for substantial improvements in access, utilization, and health status for millions of low-income Americans.

Expanded Coverage   Since the enactment of Medicare and Medicaid, there has been intermittent interest in programs to expand coverage either incrementally or through a national health insurance program. During the Nixon administration, a number of bills to expand coverage were introduced and debated by the Congress. President Carter made the introduction of national health insurance one of his campaign promises. As the 1980s draw to a close, the Congress has given serious attention to proposals that would expand employer-based coverage to reduce by two-thirds the currently uninsured population. However, to date none of these initiatives has been enacted. In the meantime, as noted above, the number and proportion of non-elderly Americans without health insurance continues to increase.

Who Are the Uninsured?

Despite the substantial improvements achieved by the Medicare and Medicaid programs, as many as 37 million nonelderly Americans were without health insurance in 1986. As shown in figure 6-1, nearly one-third of the uninsured have incomes below the federally defined poverty level, one-third have incomes between 100 and 200 percent of the poverty level, and the rest have incomes above 200 percent of the poverty level. In 1986 the federal poverty line for a family of four was $11,612.

Children under the age of eighteen make up one-third of the uninsured population. Forty percent of these children live in families with incomes below the poverty level. These children are not covered by the Medicaid program, because they live in families that do not meet the state's eligibility criteria for the Aid to Families with Dependent Children program: their households assets are too high; they live in families with two parents; they live in families with an unemployed parent in a state that does not cover these families; or the state's payment standard is considerably below the poverty level. In 1980 the percentage of children living in poverty who were not covered by Medicaid ranged from 26 percent in Washington D.C., to 80 percent in Wyoming (Johnson, Rosenbaum, and Simons, 1985).

Many people without health insurance live in families where the head of the household is employed (figure 6-2). Of adults who are uninsured, nearly 60 percent are employed on a full-time or part-time basis, 9 percent have retired early or are disabled, and another 6.5 percent are attending school. The probability of insurance coverage varies both by status of employment (steadily employed, full time, part time, nonworkers) and type of employment. Full-time, steadily employed workers and their dependents, for example, are more likely to be insured than full-year, part-time workers (87.3 percent and 67.8 percent, respectively). The disparity is even greater when looking at employer-sponsored health insurance, with 80.6 percent of full-time steadily employed workers and their families covered, but only 35.6 percent of full-year part-time workers and their families covered. The

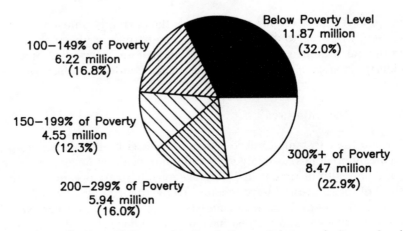

Figure 6-1.   The Nonaged Uninsured by Family Income Relative to the Poverty Level, 1987
   Source: Swartz, 1988. Reprinted by permission of the author.

rate of employer-based coverage by type of industry ranges from a low of 50.3 percent for those in personal services to 88.6 percent for persons in mining (Employee Benefit Research Institute, 1987).

Access, Utilization, and Health Status

Studies have consistently shown that access to the health care system is strongly influenced by health insurance and cost sharing (Newhouse et al., 1981; Phelps and Newhouse, 1976). Even when medical conditions and health status are about the same, persons without health insurance use fewer health services than persons with health insurance (Monheit, Hagan, and Berk, 1985). It is therefore not surprising that the implementation of both the Medicare and the Medicaid programs was accompanied by an increase in the use of health care services by the poor and the elderly. Table 6-2 presents recent information on hospital utilization rates for people with and without insurance. Although factors other than health insurance can account for some of the differences in hospitalization rates, insurance coverage is an important determinant.

   Little is known about how services are used or about the range of services used by the uninsured after they gain entry into the hospital sector. The intensity of services and their costs may be relatively low for the uninsured. Uninsured persons may avoid treatment to

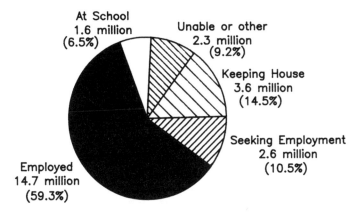

Figure 6-2.   The Labor Force Status of the Nonaged Uninsured, 1987
  Source: Swartz, 1988. Reprinted by permission of the author.

avoid significant out-of-pocket expenses. At the same time, hospitals
and physicians may render fewer services because they suspect that
they will not be paid. Either scenario creates an incentive for people
without insurance to postpone seeking care. If and when the uninsured
finally enter the medical system, they may be more likely than others
to need extensive hospital resources.

Studies of service use have reached mixed conclusions. Investigators from the Rand Corporation found that access to the health care
system was affected by cost-sharing but that once people had entered
the system there was very little difference in the use of services (Lohr
et al., 1986). Davis and Rowland (1983) found that people with health
insurance were hospitalized more days than their uninsured counterparts. Once hospitalized, insured adults between ages fifteen and forty-
four had an average length of stay of 5.1 days, self-paying patients
stayed 4.5 days, and no-charge patients were discharged after 4.4 days.

Recent surveys by the Robert Wood Johnson Foundation suggest
that lack of insurance deters people from seeking needed medical care.
According to the 1983 survey, 15 percent of uninsured families, compared with 4.8 percent of insured families, stated that they needed
medical care in 1982 but did not receive it. The families that needed
but did not receive medical services reported that financial concerns
were the main obstacle to their receiving care. In addition, an estimated one million families reported that they were refused medical
care because they could not afford to pay for treatment (Robert Wood
Johnson Foundation, 1982). The subsequent survey by the Robert
Wood Johnson Foundation in 1986 generated similar results, with 6

Table 6-2.   Hospitalization Rates by Age Group, 1980

Group	Percentage
Under age 65, with private insurance	13.5
Under age 65, with Medicaid	24.2
Under age 65, without insurance	7.1
Age 65 and older, with Medicare	39.5
Age 65 and older, without Medicare	7.6
National average	17.2

Source: Based on data from U.S. Department of Health and Human Services, 1981c.

percent of the sample, representing 13.5 million persons, reporting that they did not receive medical services for financial reasons, and approximately 1 million individuals reporting that they tried but failed to get the medical care they needed (Freeman et al., 1987).

In addition to the concern about access to care by the uninsured, there is also concern that persons without health insurance do not get treated in the most appropriate setting. For example, current policy practices may inadvertently create incentives for sick uninsured people to go to hospital emergency rooms for treatment, when physician or clinic services would be equally if not more effective and probably less costly. When the 1982–86 hospitalization rates for uninsured people were compared to those for insured individuals, the insured had higher hospitalization rates than the uninsured at both points in time, but the gap between the two groups narrowed over time, from 39 to 19 percent. During that same time period, a comparison of physician visits by uninsured and insured people documents that the difference between the groups widened significantly, from 19 to 27 percent (Freeman et al., 1987). This shift in utilization rates suggests that it may be easier for poor and uninsured persons to be admitted to a hospital than to be treated by a physician in an office.

The Distribution of Uncompensated Care

Although people without health insurance tend to have lower hospitalization rates and shorter lengths of stay than those with health insurance, many uninsured and underinsured persons nonetheless require and use hospital services. The uncompensated care costs that result from lack of insurance are neither randomly nor evenly distributed across hospitals. This is attributable in large part to two factors. First, a significant fraction of any hospital's inpatient population comes from the community in which the hospital is located, and communities vary in affluence and insurance coverage. Second, some hospitals have a strong mission to serve the poor. Many are public hospitals explicitly established for this purpose.

Data on the actual cost of uncompensated care incurred by specific hospitals are not available. One proxy for estimating uncompensated care is the proportion of hospital admissions not covered by insurance. We divide uninsured admissions into self-pay, no charge, reduced charge, and Hill-Burton patients. According to a 1981 Office of Civil Rights survey of all general short-term hospitals in the United States, uninsured admissions represented 7.3 percent of all admissions (U.S. Department of Health and Human Services, 1981a). However, there was significant variation in the extent to which hospitals admitted uninsured patients. As shown in figure 6-3, uninsured admissions accounted for less than 5 percent of total admissions in nearly half (47 percent) of all hospitals, but more than 20 percent of all admissions in 5.4 percent of hospitals.

We can examine longitudinal data for 1981 and 1986 to see whether the relative burden of uninsured admissions shifted over time. For this analysis, we compared the distribution of uninsured admissions in a matched file of more than 2,400 general medical and surgical hospitals surveyed by the Office of Civil Rights in 1981 and 1986. The 1986 survey includes only those hospitals with Hill-Burton obligations (U.S. Department of Health and Human Services, 1986a). It is therefore somewhat biased, primarily because it excludes almost all investor-owned hospitals. We looked at this sample of hospitals to see whether uncompensated care admissions increased over time. For these hospitals, uninsured admissions increased on average from 8 to 10 percent of total admissions between 1981 and 1986. However, when we looked at the distribution of uninsured cases, we found that the proportion of hospitals in which uninsured admissions accounted for more than 20 percent of total admissions increased from 6 percent in 1981 to 10 percent by 1986. This suggests that an increasing number of hospitals admitted a relatively large proportion of uninsured patients.

To examine the characteristics of hospitals with a substantial uncompensated care burden, we created a disproportionate share measure for various groups of hospitals. This measure was arrived at by dividing the share of the total number of people without health insurance who were admitted by each group of hospitals by that hospital's share of total admissions. Thus if the disproportionate share index for

144

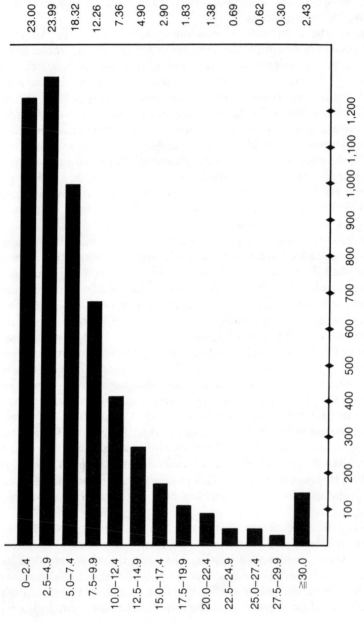

Percent of Hospitals

0–2.4	23.00
2.5–4.9	23.99
5.0–7.4	18.32
7.5–9.9	12.26
10.0–12.4	7.36
12.5–14.9	4.90
15.0–17.4	2.90
17.5–19.9	1.83
20.0–22.4	1.38
22.5–24.9	0.69
25.0–27.4	0.62
27.5–29.9	0.30
≥30.0	2.43

Uninsured as Percent of Total Admissions

Frequency

100 200 300 400 500 600 700 800 900 1,000 1,100 1,200

Figure 6.3. The Distribution of Uninsured Patients among Hospitals
Source: U.S. Department of Health and Human Services, 1981a.

a group of hospitals was over one, those hospitals treated a disproportionate share of the uninsured. The hospital groups we chose to examine are based on the characteristics that have been identified in the literature as being associated with problems of uncompensated care.

Table 6-3 reports disproportionate share measures for various categories of hospitals. Public hospitals—public teaching hospitals, in particular—admitted a larger share of uninsured admissions than hospitals in any other category. Nonteaching proprietary hospitals had the lowest proportion of uninsured admissions. Hospitals in the South provided the highest proportion of care to people without insurance (possibly because Medicaid eligibility rules are more restrictive there). It is important to point out that the findings conceal significant variation within groups. For example, not all public hospitals provided a disproportionate amount of uncompensated care: in 26.5 percent of public COTH hospitals, the uninsured made up less than 10 percent of total admissions. Likewise, not all proprietary nonteaching hospitals provided care to a relatively small proportion of uninsured patients. Uninsured patients represented more than 10 percent of total admissions in 11.3 percent of proprietary nonteaching hospitals.

In general, our findings about the distribution of uncompensated care admissions, based upon the relative number of uninsured admissions, are consistent with those of other researchers. While other researchers have used different proxies to measure the uncompensated care burden, such as the ratio of gross patient revenues, their findings about the distribution of the burden of uncompensated care across hospitals are similar to ours (Sulvetta, 1985; Sloan, Valvona, and Mullner, 1986; Commonwealth Task Force, 1985).

The Cost of Uncompensated Care

The term uncompensated care costs is a misnomer. Uncompensated care is not a cost; it is, more accurately, a deduction from revenues. However, we use the term here, because it is so widely accepted. In the previous section, we used the proportion of uninsured admissions as a proxy for the amount of uncompensated care rendered by hospitals. However, the proportion of uninsured patients treated is not an accurate indicator of actual uncompensated care costs experienced by any given hospital. Uncompensated care, by definition, is care provided by the hospital for which it does not get paid in full.

Table 6-3.   Hospitals' Share of the Uninsured, by Type of Hospital and Region, 1981

Hospital Type and Region	Total Admissions (A)	Percentage of Uninsured Admissions (B)	B/A
Public			
Major COTH	2.37	8.45	3.57
Minor COTH	0.74	2.21	2.99
Other teaching	3.62	11.51	3.18
Nonteaching	14.77	16.78	1.14
Nonprofit			
Major COTH	2.64	2.27	0.86
Minor COTH	10.79	9.37	0.87
Other teaching	20.96	15.42	0.74
Nonteaching	34.64	27.66	0.80
Proprietary			
Other teaching	0.07	0.12	1.70
Nonteaching	9.33	6.26	0.67
Region			
Northeast	21.28	15.68	0.87
North Central	28.16	19.10	0.68
West	15.86	17.65	1.11
South	34.60	44.57	1.29

Source: Based on data from U.S. Department of Health and Human Services, 1981a.

Note: In 1981 there were no proprietary major or minor COTH hospitals and only nine "other teaching" proprietary hospitals.

One definition of uncompensated care is the cost of providing hospital services to people who cannot be expected to pay for their own hospital care. A second and more controversial definition of uncompensated care is the cost of care for people who are recipients of public programs, such as Medicaid, whose rates do not cover fully the costs incurred. These costs could include uncovered days and the provision of services for which hospitals are not reimbursed. The cost of underfunded patients is even more controversial, since some unreimbursed costs may reflect, in the eyes of the payors, inefficient services.

Another definitional problem occurs when one considers public hospitals, which admit a relatively high proportion of patients without insurance. Yet these hospitals receive public subsidies to cover their deficits, deficits which result in large part because these hospitals admit people who cannot pay for their hospital care. There seems to be some disagreement as to whether these costs should be included in aggregate estimates of uncompensated care. If we are concerned about the cost of taking care of the poor and uninsured, then the costs incurred by these state and local governments should be included; if instead we are concerned about the costs for which hospitals are not paid, then they should be omitted from aggregate estimates of uncompensated care.

Despite definitional problems, a number of attempts have been made to estimate the cost of uncompensated care. An approach frequently employed measures the cost of uncompensated care as the difference between the hospital's total charges and net patient revenues. This approach, however, may be misleading: in most hospitals a relatively small proportion of patients actually pays charges, so a hospital could inflate its estimate of uncompensated care simply by raising charges (see chapter 3). Two hospitals could experience the same costs and net revenues, but the hospital with a higher markup will appear to have the greater uncompensated care costs.

The American Hospital Association (1987a) estimated that the total cost of uncompensated care was $7 billion in 1986. The figure was based upon charge-based estimates (deductions from revenues) reported by hospitals for charity care patients. Of this total, AHA estimated that tax appropriations to hospitals covered approximately $1.2 billion, leaving approximately $5.8 billion in nonreimbursed costs.

Financing Uncompensated Care

Three major sources of revenue are available to hospitals to cover uncompensated care costs. These include philanthropic contributions, cross-subsidies, and government appropriations. Recently, several financing schemes, such as disproportionate share adjustments and risk-pool allocations, have been enacted.

Philanthropy

While charitable contributions have historically been an important source of hospital revenues, the percentage of hospital income obtained through philanthropy has declined steadily. In 1903, charitable contributions accounted for 27 percent of total hospital revenues. By 1935, charitable contributions as a percentage of total revenues had declined to 14 percent. With the implementation of the Medicare and Medicaid programs, philanthropic support for hospital services decreased even further; and by 1985, philanthropy represented less than

Table 6-4.   Charge-Shifting Potential, by Type of Hospital (percent)

Ratio of Charge-Based to Uninsured Patients	Public Hospitals			
	Urban, COTH	Urban, Non-COTH, Teaching	Urban, Nonteaching	Rural
Less than 1.0	52.2	33.3	6.0	5.9
1.1–4.99	40.6	34.6	42.0	47.0
Greater than 5.0	7.2	32.0	52.0	47.0

Sources: Based on data from American Hospital Association, A, 1985; U.S. Department of Health and Human Services, 1981a.

1.3 percent of funds used for hospital care (Anderson, 1986). Barring a major change in giving, private donations are unlikely to support uncompensated care completely.

Cross-Subsidization

The most common way for hospitals to cover the costs of uncompensated care is to increase the price charged to private paying patients. This is often referred to as cost shifting, suggesting that hospitals are shifting the costs of uncompensated care from uninsured to insured patients. This term is somewhat misleading, and more appropriate terms might be *payment differential* or *revenue shifting* (Ginsberg and Sloan, 1984). Whatever it is called, hospitals have traditionally generated revenues from private patients to cover the costs of treating the uninsured.

The extent to which hospitals can and do generate revenues from private, paying patients to cover services that are not self-supporting is widely debated. According to the Health Insurance Association of America (1987), in 1985 cross-subsidies covered $3.9 billion attributable to charity care and bad debt. Other studies have confirmed the payment differential paid by commercial insurers but have cast doubt on the assumption that these higher payments are related directly to the cost of care for the uninsured and underinsured.

While raising charges for commercially insured patients is one way to cover uncompensated costs, several studies have found that the markups paid by commercial insurers do not rise or fall systematically with the individual hospital's percentage of charity care or bad debt. Hospitals able to increase charges to private paying patients do so, but the increases appear to have no direct relationship to the hospital's uncompensated care burden (Wilensky, 1986; Hadley and Feder, 1985).

	Not-for-Profit Hospitals			For-Profit Hospitals	
Urban, COTH	Urban, Non-COTH, Teaching	Urban, Nonteaching	Rural	Urban	Rural
4.6	4.2	3.7	4.6	6.0	3.4
39.0	26.9	26.0	43.0	15.8	36.9
56.2	69.0	70.3	52.7	80.6	59.6

This discrepancy may exist because hospitals with the largest share of uninsured patients have a small proportion of charge-based payors. In Table 6-4, we look at the ratio of charge-based to uninsured patients to see the extent to which hospitals in various categories would be able to use revenues from charge-based patients to subsidize care for the uninsured. The table shows that hospitals with the greatest need to cross-subsidize (public teaching hospitals, for example) are at a comparative disadvantage. From this table, it appears that these hospitals would have to increase charges substantially to a small number of paying patients to cover bad debts. Hospitals with a relatively small share of uninsured admissions (such as private, investor-owned, urban-based hospitals) have the highest ratio of charge-based to uninsured patients.

Government Appropriations

A third source of funds is a public appropriation to hospitals that incur operating deficits resulting from the provision of uncompensated care. Recently, these funds have been earmarked primarily for public facilities. Total expenditures by state and local governments to support public hospitals were $7.3 billion in 1985 (Health Care Financing Administration). In some states, public appropriations have not kept pace with the levels of bad debt and charity care experienced by public hospitals (Reed, Cawley, and Anderson, 1986).

Uncompensated Care and Financial Indicators

Current data indicate that existing financing efforts do not cover the cost of uncompensated care. One study of the relationship between uncompensated care and a hospital's financial status found that measures of liquidity, profitability, and capital structure fell as the amount of uncompensated care rose (Sloan, Valvona, and Mullner, 1986). A second study reported a similar relationship between operating deficits and uncompensated care burden (Sulvetta, 1985).

A third study investigated the total margins in different groups of hospitals. Findings showed that total margins (net revenues minus expenses as a percentage of net revenues) were lower in those groups of hospitals that provided larger amounts of uncompensated care. For example, 45 percent of public teaching hospitals had a negative total margin, compared with 26.2 percent of public nonteaching hospitals, 19.5 percent of private teaching hospitals, and 15.9 percent of private nonteaching hospitals (Commonwealth Task Force, 1985).

Control of Uncompensated Care

By most accounts, the demand for charity care and the total amount of uncompensated care delivered by hospitals has been increasing. At the same time, the changing economic environment may make it more difficult for hospitals to provide medical care to all charity care patients. These changes have triggered new initiatives to reduce the exposure of hospitals to the liability of uncompensated care.

Some believe that hospitals are modifying admitting practices and patient care practices in response to the changing economic environment (Sloan, Valvonza, and Mullner, 1986). While it is not clear that hospitals have adopted these measures in direct response to rising uncompensated care costs, it is clear that particular actions could result in limited access of the uninsured. During 1981 and 1982, nearly 15 percent of hospitals surveyed adopted explicit limits on the amount of charity care they provided. Included in this category were 26 percent of public COTH hospitals. Nearly 10 percent of hospitals surveyed reduced hours of operation or staffing in the outpatient departments, and 6 percent reduced the hours of operation in the emergency room. Both outpatient and emergency room services are considered entry points for the uninsured to inpatient services.

One of the most serious implications of the changing economic environment is the possibility that patients are being denied services because they are unable to pay for them. For example, there are reports of hospitals refusing to treat uninsured patients who cannot pay or requiring a sometimes sizable deposit prior to an admission. There are also reports about inappropriate patient transfers and patient dumping (U.S. Senate, 1985; Schiff et al., 1986). While these problems have not been evaluated systematically on a national basis and are largely anecdotal, there is nonetheless mounting evidence that seriously ill patients without insurance have been refused treatment by hospitals (Wrenn, 1985; Relman, 1985).

Antidumping Sanctions

Texas was the first state to respond to reports of inappropriate patient transfers. According to Texas statute, patients are protected against a transfer predicated upon "arbitrary, capricious, or unreasonable discrimination based upon race, religion, national origin, age, sex, physical condition or economic status" (State of Texas, 1987).

The Congress has also enacted antidumping legislation in response to numerous reports of inappropriate transfers. The Consolidated Omnibus Budget Reconciliation Act of 1985 forbids hospitals to transfer patients who are in a medically unstable condition or in active labor unless specified prerequisites have been met. The receiving hospital, for example, must now agree to the transfer and have the space and personnel to treat the patient properly. The transferring hospital must certify in writing that the medical benefits outweigh the risks associated with the transfer. If hospitals fail to comply with the new law, which is designed to protect medically unstable uninsured persons, numerous sanctions may be applied.

Compensating Hospitals for Charity Care Costs

The term level the playing field has been applied to hospital compensation, suggesting that all hospitals can compete equally if an alternative source of paying them for caring for uninsured patients can be found. This can be done by using a variety of approaches, including indigent care pools, rate-setting programs, and disproportionate share adjustments.

Indigent care pools require states to collect revenues from a variety of sources and then to redistribute the funds to hospitals based on the amount of bad debt and charity care provided. Some states raise funds for the pool through a tax on hospital revenues. New York State, for example, requires that hospitals make payments (based on their net revenues) into a pool, from which allocations are made to hospitals that admit a significant proportion of uninsured patients. This approach perpetuates the practice of cross-subsidization, because patient revenues are taxed to finance care for uninsured patients (Lewin and Lewin, 1987). With indigent care pools, states can attempt to level the playing field: funds can be used to compensate hospitals for providing charity care in a price-competitive market.

Rate setting is another approach. States with rate-setting programs allow higher reimbursement rates for those hospitals that provide a significant amount of uncompensated care. For example, Maryland takes the approach of building the costs of uncompensated care into each hospital's rate. To the extent that all payors pay the same rate, all payors contribute equally to cover the costs of treating uninsured patients in hospitals throughout the state.

Disproportionate share adjustments is a third approach. For example, Medicare and Medicaid programs currently allow adjustments in payments to hospitals for uncompensated care. When these programs were first implemented, hospital reimbursement rates were based on retrospective cost-based reimbursement. This meant that bad debts, other than those incurred directly by program beneficiaries, were not recognized as allowable costs. That policy has been changed.

The implementation of the Medicare prospective payment system in 1983 triggered concern that Medicare payment levels would threaten the financial position of hospitals that provided a disproportionate share of services to low-income patients. However, there were two competing, never clearly differentiated, policy initiatives being promoted. The first was that Medicare should help subsidize the cost of all uncompensated care; the second was that low-income Medicare patients were more costly to treat and that the DRG payment rates should be adjusted accordingly. The resolution incorporates both views in the payment formula.

With respect to Medicaid, Congress passed legislation in 1981 which gave the states greater latitude in designing their hospital payment systems (Section 2173 of the Omnibus Budget Reconciliation Act of 1981). The legislation required that the new payment levels (1) be reasonable and adequate to meet the costs of efficiently and economically operated facilities, (2) assure access to Medicaid patients, and (3) take into account the circumstances of hospitals that serve a disproportionate number of low-income patients.

Expanding Insurance Coverage

As a result of the problems associated with uncompensated care, there has been increased legislative activity in expanding coverage to reduce the number of uninsured persons. The federal government is exploring a variety of options, and a number of states have enacted policies and are considering new proposals to decrease the number of people without health insurance. Washington State for example, recently adopted a proposal that makes health insurance available to poor uninsured people. Other states have established risk pools to provide insurance to the so-called medically uninsurable people (those who have medical conditions that are not covered under standard policies) and have engaged in efforts to decrease the cost of insurance to small groups. Many states have opted to expand eligibility through the Medicaid program.

Federal Initiatives   In 1985, the Congress enacted legislation that requires employers with health insurance plans to continue offering coverage to former employees and their dependents for eighteen months (if the worker becomes unemployed or works fewer hours) and for thirty-six months to dependents of deceased workers. In 1986, the Congress adopted a provision to expand Medicaid benefits to address the problems of uninsured women and children. This new law gives states the option of extending benefits to infants and children up to age five in two-parent families with an income below a state's poverty level. The provision would also extend coverage of prenatal and postnatal services to these families. States have the option of partially or fully revising their eligibility criteria. If all states were to extend benefits fully, the number of uninsured could be reduced by as much as 40 percent (Children's Defense Fund, 1988). To date, nearly half of all states have responded to the 1986 law.

Recently, there has been a great deal of interest in Congress to decrease the number of uninsured Americans by mandating employers to offer health insurance to employees. During 1988, the Senate Labor and Human Resources Committee reported out the Minimum Health Benefits for All Workers Act of 1988, which had the following key components:

1. Employers would be required to provide all full-time employees (people who work a minimum of 17.5 hours per week) and their dependents (excluding those already with coverage) with health insurance;
2. Employers (including those already offering insurance to employees) would have to meet specified minimum standards (e.g., they must include certain benefits such as prenatal care);
3. Each plan would have a maximum annual deductible as established by Congress and maximum out-of-pocket costs.

Proponents of this approach argue that it would extend coverage to some 23 million persons who are now uninsured (U.S. Congress, Congressional Budget Office, 1987).

State Initiatives   The Massachusetts program, enacted in April 1988, initially encourages and ultimately requires all employers with five or more employees to offer health insurance to full-time employees; it established minimum benefits for all employer-sponsored health benefits programs. Employers contribute to a state fund to help finance the cost of insuring employees and workers receiving unemployment compensation. Employers who already provide health coverage to employees can deduct the cost of the insurance from the new state surcharge. Firms with six or fewer employees will be able to join a newly created insurance pool for small businesses to help finance the cost of health insurance. The new program is expected to extend health insurance coverage to 600,000 currently uninsured individuals. New York State, also focused on employment-related loss of coverage, recently decided to help pay health insurance premiums on a short-term basis for workers who have lost their jobs as a result of plant closings. Oregon has decided to offer tax credits to employers that provide insurance to previously uninsured workers (Pear, 1987).

Washington State has established a program designed to extend health coverage to uninsured persons living in families with incomes up to 200 percent of the federal poverty level. The program is to be financed by general revenues and an income-based premium. Payment to providers is on a capitated basis. Providers assume a portion of the risk for managing the care for the newly covered population. The program begins in five geographic regions and is expected to include approximately 30,000 residents.

Many states have revised Medicaid eligibility criteria to include a greater portion of low-income uninsured adults and their dependents. Nearly half of all states include additional pregnant women and children, in response to recent changes in Title XIX. Minnesota, for example, revised its Medicaid eligibility criteria, providing copayments for pregnant women and for children under age six who live in low-income families. Rhode Island covers poor children up to age eighteen who live in two-parent families.

The states are using a variety of financing schemes to fund expansions in coverage. Both Florida and South Carolina tax hospital revenues to finance Medicaid expansions. Other states rely upon general revenues and revenues obtained from an increase in the cigarette tax. States have also tried to increase the number of individuals with health insurance by lowering the cost of insurance. Over fifteen states have created risk pools that offer coverage to otherwise uninsurable persons.

Risk Pools Some states have established quasi-public risk pools to finance and extend coverage to the uninsured. The uninsured can purchase health insurance through risk pools jointly financed by government, employer, and consumer contributions. While the characteristics of risk pools vary across the states, they have a number of common features. They are financed by both general tax revenues and funds raised from insurance companies, so that the cost of decreasing the number of uninsured is shared by the public and private sectors.

Typically, a board of trustees is formed to organize a statewide consortium of health insurance companies. The board, working with insurers, develops a standard policy with defined benefits, eligibility criteria, premium rates, and maximum copayments. Many states require insurance companies to share the cost of the annual deficit incurred by the pools. As of 1985, all but one state pool sold health insurance exclusively to the medically uninsurable population (Bovbjerg and Koller, 1986).

The risk-pool model has considerable appeal: the cost of administering the plan is low if enough people enroll so that it can take advantage of economies of scale, and it offers health insurance coverage to people who would otherwise be unable to obtain it. The insurance industry has generally supported this approach.

In practice, the pools have not been successful in decreasing the numbers of the uninsured. The most serious problems arise because, in all but one state, coverage is restricted to the medically uninsurable. Adverse selection is therefore built in, bringing along problems of high costs, high premiums (premiums are more than 125 percent above the cost of comparable plans), low enrollments, and increasing deficits. In the past, many private health insurance companies have resisted proposals to allow the state to enroll people who otherwise would have purchased insurance from them. Many eligible uninsured persons have not enrolled in state plans because they either cannot afford the premium or are unaware that the plan exists.

To improve the success of the pools, many states are looking at ways to increase enrollment and to bring more of the eligible population into the pool. A Connecticut plan has just begun to enroll all uninsured persons, not just the medically uninsurables, to introduce greater economies of scale, minimize the increase in premiums, and reduce adverse selection (Bovbjerg and Koller, 1986). With a larger pool of enrollees, including the relatively healthy uninsured population, many believe that the pool model could become self-supporting and could offer coverage to a larger portion of the uninsured population (Mulstein, 1984). As of December 1987, fifteen states have created insurance pools.

Medicaid Buy-In   Proposals to allow individuals to buy coverage from the Medicaid program have been put forth in recent years. The public cost of such a program could vary depending upon the level of public support for poor, near poor, and other uninsured persons. Premiums could be paid on a sliding-scale basis, allowing the value of the government subsidy to decrease as the individual's income and contribution increases. This approach could build upon the structure of employer-provided health insurance and at the same time expand the public role to help support poor, uninsured, and newly unemployed individuals. It would use the existing Medicaid financing and delivery system to offer coverage and services to the uninsured population.

In many ways, states are taking the lead in an effort to limit the number of uninsured Americans. Despite these initiatives, the number of uninsured Americans continues to increase. Without a more comprehensive solution, the problems of the uninsured and the related problems of uncompensated care are likely to persist in the years ahead.

part III | Policy
Options

In the remaining four chapters, we present a series of recommendations. We propose modifications to the hospital payment system for inpatient care, a major revision in the financing of clinical education, minor revisions in the financing of clinical research, and a new system for covering the uninsured.

In generating these policy recommendations, we developed a series of general principles. We believe that general principles are necessary to ensure that the proposed recommendations are consistent across the four services. In the past, there has been a tendency to focus upon only one service, possibly because of the difficulty of reconciling the differences between various services and of merging various types of recommendations into a consistent policy. This book attempts to apply a consistent approach to policy reform for each service.

The first principle is that services, not hospitals, are of primary concern. Recent public policy discussions tend to focus on how well individual hospitals or groups of hospitals are doing. Legislation has allowed hospitals with a large commitment to clinical education or to charity care to receive additional payments, an adjustment designed primarily to maintain the financial solvency of the particular hospitals. Only indirectly do the initiatives support the services themselves.

A second principle is that the current level of service is not necessarily appropriate or even desirable. Earlier financial arrangements may have led to too much of some services, to too few of others, or to services of the wrong type. For each service it is necessary first to consider the appropriate level needed, to review the incentives created by the current system, and to modify the incentives to meet policy objectives.

A third principle is that marketplace solutions should be used whenever possible. This recognizes that the health care system is becoming more competitive and that solutions that are contrary to the marketplace will be very difficult to implement. It recognizes, for example, that cross-subsidization cannot continue indefinitely.

A fourth principle is that the provision of certain services will require government intervention. Public support will be necessary to subsidize those services that are not self-financing but are deemed to serve a worthwhile social function. In addition, government regulation may be necessary to ensure the supply and quality of a given service.

chapter 7 | Patient Care

As discussed in chapter 2, approximately 90 percent of the revenues hospitals receive for providing patient care services comes from third parties; that is, government programs and insurance plans that make payments on behalf of their beneficiaries and enrollees. Before 1980, most third parties paid hospitals either their billed charges (or some percentage thereof) or made payments based on estimates of the costs the hospitals actually incurred in rendering services to program beneficiaries. These reimbursement mechanisms usually enabled hospitals to recover the full costs they incurred in taking care of insured patients and frequently resulted in small operating surpluses. Surpluses from patient care were often used to subsidize the cost of providing hospital services to the uninsured and to support clinical education and biomedical research.

The changes in hospital payment systems implemented in the early 1980s have fundamentally changed hospitals' financial environments. Hospitals now face substantial financial risk; that is, they can make large profits or losses on patient care services. These profits and losses can occur at the hospital level (i.e., the hospitals' net operating margins can be positive or negative), at the level of an insured group (Medicare, Medicaid), or at the patient level (patients with certain characteristics are winners, other are losers).

In chapter 2 we noted that, although hospital profit levels had reached historic highs during the first two years of the prospective payment system (PPS), hospital profits have started to fall, and profits of the average hospital are expected to be negative by 1990. Since this situation is without precedent, it is difficult to predict how hospital decision makers will respond to it. We expect, however, that patients whose costs are not fully covered by the payment system are especially vulnerable in the changing health care environment. These patients may have difficulty receiving all of the services they require, if hospitals are not adequately paid for caring for them. It is important to determine why the payments that hospitals receive for taking care of patients may not cover the cost of the care provided. Is it caused by imperfections in the payment system or by the actions of the hospital? If the problem is caused by the design of the payment system, the policy response should be to modify the way payment rates are set.

In this chapter, we review methods of establishing hospital payments for patient care services and make recommendations for modifying these methods. We begin the chapter with a brief statement of goals that should guide policy decisions. The remainder of the chapter is divided into two sections. The first section suggests reforms to prospective payment systems, with most of the attention given to the Medicare prospective payment system. The discussion of these reforms is further divided into two steps; reforms that propose changes in the method for setting the overall payment level to hospitals (step one) and reforms that suggest specific adjustments to the system that may reduce the vulnerability of patients who are high cost relative to other patients in their payment category (step two). The second section discusses the competitive approaches and how they can be modified to take into account differences in the cost of treating the average patient (step three) and the high-cost patient (step four).

Policy Goals

We assume that the major goals guiding policy makers who are implementing or modifying prospective payments systems are (1) to develop payment systems that control the growth in hospital expenditures, (2) to promote the efficient delivery of hospital services, and (3) to ensure beneficiaries access to covered health care services of appropriate quality. The terms efficient, access, and appropriate quality are value laden; nevertheless, they do provide some guidance for policy makers. For example, if the goal is to promote access to care for all beneficiaries, then the payment system should be designed toward that end. Hospitals should not be given financial incentives to discriminate against certain groups of beneficiaries. Further, efficiently managed hospitals, which because of their geographic location or some other factor outside of their control, should receive payments adequate to deliver care of appropriate quality.

The access criterion also suggests that the effect of the payment system on patients' travel and time costs should be explicitly taken into consideration. An implication of this is that people should be able to receive hospital care in their own communities. There are obvious exceptions to this statement. In general, local hospitals must be able to provide care of acceptable quality. Second, to provide specific services (such as open-heart surgery), hospitals must have sufficient volume of cases to maintain quality. Third, for some services (such as organ transplants), it may be most efficient to deliver care in national or regional centers. In addition to these goals, another important policy goal is to develop a system that seems fair in its treatment of different hospitals and that is not too costly to implement.

Prospective Payment System Reform

Step One

Modify prospective payment systems to recognize explicitly more of the factors that explain why one hospital is more expensive than another. The average hospital now receives over half of its revenues from third parties which pay on the basis of prospectively set rates. The Medicare program, some state Medicaid programs, several state rate-setting commissions, and certain Blue Cross plans all use this general approach, although the rate-setting methods vary considerably.

In this section, we focus on the Medicare prospective payment system, for several reasons. First, many of the problems that arise in the Medicare program's prospective payment system are representative of generic problems that occur in all programs. Second, the Medicare program covers the single largest group of patients and is responsible for over one-third of patient care revenues in most hospitals. Third, designers of all prospective payment systems must decide which of the particular factors influencing hospital costs they will take into account in setting rates. Since the Medicare program establishes payment rates for inpatient care rendered by almost all hospitals across the United States, the design of its prospective payment system offers a greater methodological challenge than state-level systems.

Under the Medicare prospective payment system, only a small number of factors are taken into consideration in setting the payment rates for a particular hospital (chapters 2 and 3). Under PPS, the payment that a hospital receives depends primarily on the hospital's standardized costs and the DRG into which the patient is classified. If the patient is an exceptionally long-stay or costly patient, the hospital will receive outlier payments. Other factors that affect the hospital's payment include the size of its graduate medical education program (the adjustment for the indirect costs of graduate medical education) and the proportion of its population on Medicaid (the adjustment for disproportionate share of low-income patients). In making recommendations for changing PPS, we focus specifically on issues related to the definition of standardized cost, case mix classification, and outlier policy. The allowance for indirect medical education and disproportionate share are discussed in chapters 8 and 10, respectively.

Recommendation One: Core Counties   Medicare should redefine the geographic areas for which it calculates the hospital wage index used in adjusting the national rate to take into consideration relative differences in labor costs. Specifically, it should divide the metropolitan statistical area (MSA) into a core county and the surrounding counties that make up the MSA and create three geographic regions (urban, suburban, rural).

A major determinant of the hospital's payment under PPS is its standardized cost. The standardized cost is based on the average national Medicare hospital cost per discharge. National rates are calculated separately for urban and rural areas. In urban areas, the urban national cost per discharge is adjusted for differences in wage levels paid to hospital workers in the MSA in which the hospital is located, while in rural areas, the rural national rate is adjusted for the relative wage differences paid to workers in the rural areas in the state in which the hospital is located. The current payment differential between urban and rural areas is more than ten percent. Frequently, these geographic areas are not good proxies for the hospital labor market area for particular hospitals. For example, the Chicago MSA includes Cook County, DuPage County, and McHenry County. It is highly unlikely that hospitals in the suburban areas operate in the same labor market as hospitals in the city of Chicago.

Researchers have shown that labor costs are often substantially higher in the core counties than in the ring counties of the MSA (Ashby, 1984). Analyses of hospital cost functions indicate that (after explicitly controlling for other factors) hospital costs are 12 percent higher in the core counties of MSAs with over 1 million people (Anderson and Lave, 1986). If this variation is not accounted for, then as payment rates are tightened, hospitals in high-cost areas will be increasingly penalized, not because they are inefficient but because they incur higher labor costs. We propose, therefore, that three categories be created—urban, suburban, and rural—instead of simply urban and rural.

The major drawback to this approach is that more payment groups will be created, which means that some hospitals will just miss being classified into a group that receives higher payments. While this result is inevitable, the creation of more groups should reduce the difference in payment rates between urban and rural hospitals.

Recommendation Two: Nonlabor Costs   Payment rates should be adjusted for regional variation in nonlabor costs as well as labor costs. Variations in the costs of energy, malpractice insurance premiums, food, and other goods and services should be taken into account explicitly. In addition, the payment rates should be adjusted for the size of the MSA in which the hospital is located.

The PPS adjusts for differences in wages, only, because labor is the only factor of production for which there are uniform data across geographic areas. However, labor costs are not the only costs that vary geographically. For example, the price of energy varies significantly across the United States. Using data from sixteen urban areas, we found that in 1986 the mean price of piped gas per 100 therms ranged from $49.30 to $84.72, with a mean of $51.56. The price of electricity per 500 kilowatt hours ranged from $32.29 to $60.07, while the price of No. 2 fuel oil ranged from $1.05 to $1.21. Prices of other goods and services purchased by hospitals may show similar variations. By not adjusting for these variations, PPS may be systematically penalizing certain hospitals and rewarding others because of their geographic location.

It will be necessary to collect new data to implement this recommendation. The data could be collected by periodically surveying a sample of hospitals to obtain information on the prices they pay for supplies. The HCFA could use these data to construct a nonlabor cost index similar to the HCFA wage index.

Recommendation Three: Rebasing   The cost information that forms the basis for the prospective payment rates should be recalculated at fixed intervals, such as every four years. National rates (as well as hospital-specific and regional rates) are based on 1981 hospital cost data, which were trended forward to set the rates in 1984. Since 1984, those rates have been increased each year by amounts established through the policy process. Although the original law indicated that the system should be rebased in the future, rebasing has not yet occurred. Rebasing explicitly recognizes changes in medical practice and the cost of treatment.

Conceptually, one can think of a prospective pricing system as a proxy for a competitive system. A price is set that reflects the estimate of the average cost of producing services. Providers have financial incentives to increase the efficiency with which services are provided, and as they respond to these incentives, the cost of care is lowered. In this case, regulators should reduce the price. On the other hand, if costs rise, then eventually regulators will have to increase the price to cover costs. Under a competitive system, prices will eventually reflect costs. This must also happen in a regulated world. Although PPS rates have been increased each year, the increases are still done in reference to 1981 data. More recent data are available and should be used.

Step Two

Modify prospective payment systems to adjust for the fact that case mix classification systems do not adequately account for differences among patients and for the fact that this may lead to discrimination against high-cost patients. Under the Medicare prospective payment system, the DRG is the unit of payment. The DRG system was originally selected because in 1982 it was the only completely developed patient classification system and because it had already been used for payment purposes. The DRG system has been modified periodically to account for improved patient data and for changing medical practice. However, the DRG classification system has been criticized because it groups together patients who are sometimes clinically dissimilar, with consequently quite different service needs. Since, with the exception of outlier payments, a hospital is paid the same amount for all patients in a DRG, some patients are winners and others are losers.

This heterogeneity has two implications. First, if some hospitals admit a higher proportion of high-cost patients within a given DRG or across many DRGs, these hospitals will incur losses, not because they are inefficient, but because they did not receive an average draw of patients. Second, high-cost patients within a DRG are losers. If the characteristics of these patients can be identified a priori, then some hospitals may try to avoid admitting them. This could reduce access for patients with certain conditions. Hospitals could also try to discharge patients earlier, thereby jeopardizing quality of care.

Recommendation Four: Case Mix Research   Continued research on the development of alternative case mix measures as well as comparative independent evaluations of these systems is necessary. Especially critical are demonstrations that use alternative case mix measures to pay hospitals. As part of a demonstration, a number of alternative case mix classification systems, which have already been developed, could be used in conjunction with (or as a replacement for) DRGs to set payment rates.

A number of researchers have proposed that other patient classification systems (severity of illness, disease staging, and MEDISGRPS) be used to modify the DRG classification system or to replace it (patient management categories). The HCFA has supported considerable research on the development of these systems as well as on the modification of the DRG system. It has also funded independent evaluations of the comparative attributes of some or all of the different systems. To date, the results of this evaluation research do not point to any clear direction for improvement (Jencks and Dobson, 1987). However, this finding may be reversed as better hospital data become available. This area is still one of critical importance.

Equally important, however, is the establishment of demonstration projects to test the implication of paying hospitals on the basis of one of the other case mix systems. A case mix classification system that looks promising on paper might have a serious defect, which is manifested only when it is used for payment purposes. New Jersey is currently testing the severity-of-illness instrument in twenty hospitals. More of these tests are necessary.

Before leaving the issue of case mix classification systems, we should point out that improvements in classification are also needed for quality of care purposes. In order to compare the quality of care across hospitals, we believe that it is necessary to have better information on the clinical condition of the patients than is incorporated in the DRGs. Thus it is possible that improvements in patient classification systems might make little difference to hospital revenues but would provide better information to hospital managers and would facilitate quality of care studies.

Recommendation Five: Proxies for Case Mix   In the short run, the HCFA should continue to use proxies for case mix complexity not accounted for by the DRGs. These proxies include the size of the graduate medical education program as measured by the resident-to-bed ratio.

The adjustment for indirect costs of graduate medical education is made to adjust for the incremental costs of clinical education and for unmeasured differences in case mix not accounted for by the DRGs. The ratio of interns and residents per bed is a convenient proxy for many of the factors associated with higher costs in teaching hospitals, many of which we cannot measure directly. Until these other factors are identified explicitly and policy decisions are made about which of them to adjust for in the PPS rates, we recommend that an adjustment for indirect medical education be retained. It should be based upon an empirically determined formula (Anderson and Lave, 1986).

Recommendation Six: Outlier Payments   The proportion of payments made as outlier payments should be increased, with all of the emphasis placed on high-cost patients and not longer-stay patients.

In addition to improving the DRG patient classification system, there are other approaches that take into account DRG patient heterogeneity. Under PPS, the hospital receives outlier payments for patients who, relative to the average patient in the DRG, are in the hospital for a long time or who incur high charges. These payments are in addition to regular PPS payments. They are designed to protect the hospital from financial risk and the patient from discrimination.

Research has indicated that, in spite of these outlier payments, hospitals still incur significant losses when treating outlier patients. In order to reduce the magnitude of the losses the hospital incurs for treating these patients, the payment to outlier cases should be increased. To this end, outlier payments for patients who meet both the length-of-stay threshold and the high-cost threshold should be paid under the high-cost rules.

A second adjustment is to pay a greater share of the total cost of the high-cost case. Currently, all cases that become outliers are money losses for the hospital. In 1986 the loss on outliers averaged over $7,000 per discharge (ProPac, 1988b). We recommend that the loss on outlier patients be reduced over time.

Discrimination against high-cost cases would be an unfortunate, unintended result of prospective payment. To be sure, countervailing pressure from physicians, arising from concerns about quality of care, professional ethics, or malpractice, as well as hospitals' interests in maintaining a reputation for high-quality medicine, decreases the likelihood that such service restrictions will take place (Anderson and Steinberg, 1984b). However, this problem is potentially very serious.

Peer review organizations should be required to monitor the extent to which certain patients are vulnerable under PPS. They should monitor when patients are underserved.

Recommendation Seven: Additional Payments for Specific Categories of Patients   Patients with certain identifiable characteristics or who need certain high-cost services should be classified into separate DRGs or have an incremental amount added to their payment amount.

Although increasing the outlier payments will decrease hospital losses in treating high-cost patients, it does not eliminate them, and some patients may still be at risk under prospective payment systems. The ability of hospitals or physicians to identify patients who generate losses for hospitals raises concerns about threats to access and to quality of care. For example, hospitals could stop providing services such as parenteral nutrition and plasmapheresis (Steinberg and Anderson, 1987). Alternatively, hospital administrators could discourage physicians from admitting patients who require such services.

We propose two complementary approaches to ameliorating this situation. The first is to create additional DRGs for patients with select medical conditions, such as cystic fibrosis. The second is to add a fixed amount of the payment rate every time a patient has a specific condition or receives a certain type of service. Both of these approaches have been recommended by the Prospective Payment Assessment Commission, although they usually have not been adopted.

The implementation of these recommendations could lead to a significant increase in the number of DRG categories (approach one) or to an increase in the number of adjustments (approach two). In addition, the implementation of these recommendations might be viewed as a return to cost-based reimbursement. Thus it would be important to limit the number of exceptions to extreme cases and to develop explicit criteria for appropriate care.

Recommendation Eight: Criteria for Appropriateness   Professional associations, the Institute of Medicine, and other interested parties should develop criteria to indicate when a particular service is necessary and when it is inappropriate.

The establishment of an additional payment for patients who receive a particular service, such as parenteral nutrition, would in a sense be a return to cost-based reimbursement, a system that provided little financial incentive for hospitals or physicians to distinguish between necessary and unnecessary treatments or procedures. As a result, an adjustment in per-case payment should be tied to criteria indicating when a particular service is appropriate.

At the present time, these criteria do not exist and need to be developed. One approach would be to have the criteria developed by professional associations, which would need to demonstrate that the criteria were based on objective data. The Association for Enteral and Parenteral Nutrition (ASPEN), for example, has already developed criteria for the appropriate use of total parenteral nutrition. Third-party payors and government agencies should monitor the criteria to make sure that unnecessary procedures are indeed excluded.

Recommendation Nine: Low-Cost, Short-Stay Outlier Policy Medicare should implement a short-stay, low-cost outlier policy.

We have so far concentrated the discussion on resolving problems that may arise because some patients classified into the same DRG are much more costly to treat than others. However, the converse is also true: some patients are much less costly to treat than other patients classified into the same DRG. For example, patients who received angioplasty were originally classified in the same DRG as coronary bypass graft surgery patients. Until those patients were reclassified, hospitals received large profits on all angioplasty patients. A low-cost outlier policy would have resulted in much lower payments for treating these patients.

The establishment of a short-stay outlier policy would have an important side benefit. In a budget-neutral world, increased payments for outlier cases must be accompanied by a decrease in payments for all nonoutlier patients. If a low-cost, short-stay outlier policy is implemented, then some funds would be transferred from low-cost to high-cost patients within a given DRG.

Recommendation Ten: Pricing Studies   The HCFA should support research on the DRG price structure to determine whether it reflects the relative cost of treating patients across different DRGs.

Under PPS, each DRG is given a relative weight, which reflects the cost of treating patients in that DRG relative to the cost of treating the average patient discharged from U.S. hospitals. Concern has been expressed that the weights do not accurately reflect the relative cost of treating patients in the different DRGs; that is, the DRG price structure may be distorted (Lave, 1985). As hospitals' financial status becomes more precarious, it is likely that they—and physicians—are more likely to respond to the relative price structure. If, because of are not, hospitals will have strong financial incentives to encourage physicians to admit patients belonging to the former DRGs and to discourage admissions or perhaps encourage undertreatment in the latter. Consequently, it is important to determine whether the price structure is reasonable.

Recommendation Eleven: The Hospital-Specific Factor   To recognize the fact that PPS cannot account for all of the factors that legitimately influence hospital costs, PPS should include a fraction of the hospital's own cost in its base rate.

Although the above recommendations would be an improvement in the design of PPS, it is impossible to account for all of the factors that should be taken into consideration in setting hospital prices. The economic environments within which hospitals operate and the availability of alternative health care will influence the cost of care in given institutions and the approaches to treatment that can be considered. In spite of improved outlier policies, some hospitals will admit patients who are relatively more costly than the average in the DRGs, while others will admit those who are relatively cheaper. These patient patterns are likely to persist over time. Including a hospital-specific factor in setting the standardized rate would be a "fudge factor" to adjust for factors that are legitimate sources of cost differences but that our measurement systems are not sensitive enough to take into consideration.

The Congress has removed the hospital-specific component in setting PPS rates. However, we believe that the inclusion of a hospital-specific factor would obviate the need to fine tune the system.

Summary: Prospective Payment Systems Adjustment Factors
We realize that most of these recommendations will lead to an increase in the complexity of the Medicare PPS as well as to a redistribution of Medicare payments across hospitals. This redistribution may make some of the proposals politically infeasible, as hospitals that stand to lose Medicare dollars will lobby against their implementation. However, we believe that both the Congress and the administration are serious about controlling Medicare outlays and thus that Medicare payment rates will be tightly controlled. If this belief is correct, then it is important to adjust payment rates for those factors over which hospitals have limited control and that lead to significant differences in the cost of producing hospital services. Our recommendations are based on the assumption that the system should and will respond to

systematic patterns of profits and losses that result from differences in the nature of the patients treated or from differences in the prices that hospitals must pay for their factors of production.

Allowing Comparability in Competitive Systems

Step Three

Competitive systems should incorporate legitimate differences in case mix, input prices, and other factors in determining payment rates. The hospital sector is not a purely competitive industry. It is probably better characterized as monopolistically competitive, because each hospital offers a somewhat different product, and the consumer has incomplete information. Hospitals vary with respect to facilities, quality of care, and the nature of the care provided. Consequently, each hospital faces a downward-sloping demand curve and will be able to charge a slightly different amount for its services.

As the industry becomes more price competitive and as organizations and individuals become more sophisticated purchasers of hospital services, the nature of the demand for hospital services changes. Some product differences will be eliminated and others retained as consumers make their preferences known. We assume that better information on quality of care and measures of output will become available over time.

There are some advantages to using the market to allocate hospital services. Many issues that must be addressed if prices are set by regulation are irrelevant if prices are set by the market. For example, under PPS, explicit decisions must be made about which factors to adjust for in setting hospital rates. Under PPS, the MSA is assumed to be the relevant labor market, and the average wage rate paid by all hospitals in the MSA is assumed to be relevant for any given hospital in it. Consequently, the average MSA wage rate is used to adjust each hospital's standardized costs. The implicit assumption behind this adjustment is that the MSA is also the relevant product market. Under a market system, the issue of the relevant labor market and the relevant product market are of secondary importance, because relevant markets form naturally. For example, if people who live in downtown Chicago are unwilling to use hospitals in Gary, Indiana, or even suburban Chicago, then the prices that hospitals charge in those areas, and the prices that they must pay for their inputs, will have little influence on the prices that are set in Chicago.

For other factors, the competitive market requires additional information in order to operate efficiently.

Recommendation Twelve: Basis of Comparison   The basis for price competition should take into consideration the nature of the patients treated. The price per case type (DRGs or other case mix systems) is a better basis for competition than simply the price per day or discharge.

As buyers of care become more sophisticated, we expect that there will be more comparative shopping. Large buyers will seek to negotiate payment rates with particular hospitals. They could agree to pay a certain amount per day, per admission, or per DRG, or they could negotiate a reduction in charges. The effect will depend partly on the basis on which the competition takes place. If the negotiation is not based on similar outputs, the impact could be undesirable.

We recommend that comparisons always include an adjustment for case mix. This is equivalent to adjusting for output differences.

If case mix differences are not taken into explicit consideration in determining the basis of the price competition, then teaching and other tertiary care hospitals will have a difficult time competing for patients with more routine medical problems, who currently make up a considerable portion of all hospitals' inpatient case mix. Hospitals could have similar cost structures for those patients.

Step Four

Allow for the protection of high-cost patients in competitive systems. As the health care system becomes more competitive, it becomes increasingly likely that certain high-cost patients will become less desirable to treat. As hospitals compete on the basis of price, one or two categories of very expensive cases could reduce the hospital's profit margin substantially. This in turn could affect the hospital's competitive position.

Recommendation Thirteen: Identify High-Cost Patients   Certain patients because of their diagnosis or treatment regime are much more likely to be high-cost patients. If these patients could be identified a priori and paid under a different system, it would be possible to prevent discrimination against them and allow hospitals that treat these patients to compete in the marketplace.

This recommendation requires the development of a list of cases that are expected to be high cost. (For example, the Maryland Health Services Cost Review Commission has developed a list for Maryland hospitals.) The criteria could include the diagnosis of the patient and possibly the procedure. Separate payment systems would be developed for these cases, and hospitals could report their cost per discharge without including these patients. This recommendation is similar to the PPS proposal for outliers. It provides the hospital a possibility for relief when a catastrophic patient arrives.

chapter 8 | Clinical Education

To meet the health care needs of our nation, an adequate supply of qualified physicians is needed. Federal financing and immigration policies in the 1960s and early 1970s, targeted to increase the physician population, were successful in generating more doctors (chapter 4). In fact, data indicate that there will be a significant surplus of physicians by 1990 (U.S. Department of Health and Human Services, 1980). Although in aggregate there may be enough physicians, there is a continued maldistribution across specialties and geographical location (chapter 4). With aggregate supply needs met and possibly surpassed, a question arises of who should be responsible for deciding the future financing of clinical education and who should chart the direction.

From chapters 1 and 4 it is clear that clinical education programs add to the cost of teaching hospitals and that some of the incremental costs are attributable to graduate medical education. However, when hospital and physician costs are combined, the incremental cost of clinical education programs is much lower, since residents and other trainees appear to substitute for attending physicians. In this chapter we present a series of frequently cited rationales for financing clinical education and make specific recommendations that would change the methods of financing and controlling clinical education programs. We expect that if these changes were adopted, specialty training choices would gradually change to more accurately reflect health care needs across both specialty and geographic location.

A careful review of the methods of controlling and financing clinical education is warranted for a number of reasons. There is a concern that the current distribution of health professionals does not match national needs, and that the educational system is not responsive to the changing health care environment (Commonwealth Task Force, 1985). This is especially true of residency education, which may be training too many specialists and too few physicians in certain areas, such as geriatrics.

There is also concern that clinical education is not being responsive to evolving patterns in the delivery of health care. Students are not being trained in the type of settings where the demand for services is increasing, such as freestanding outpatient centers and health maintenance organizations. As a result, it may be necessary to increase the emphasis on training in ambulatory care settings and to decrease the training in tertiary care sites. In addition, because there is no centralized method of controlling graduate medical education programs, any change in the content of education programs is likely to be piecemeal and disjointed (Stevens, 1978).

Current Financing Methods

The financing of clinical education has become an issue of public policy concern because the method of financing hospital services has changed so dramatically in recent years. Teaching hospitals can no longer rely on cost-based and charge-based reimbursement to cover the cost of clinical education. Medicare and some Medicaid programs have explicitly identified the incremental costs of clinical education and have designed separate payment systems. Other payors have adopted a more competitive approach to setting hospital payment rates, which may or may not pay for the incremental cost of training programs. These reduced payment rates may diminish the hospital's ability to cross-subsidize clinical education.

The current financing system assumes that incremental costs and benefits are borne by the teaching hospital; thus financing arrangements have reimbursed the teaching hospital for residency education. As shown in chapters 1, 2, and 4, however, more recent data suggest that these assumptions are incorrect. The attending physician appears to benefit substantially from the presence of residents. Frequently, the resident substitutes for attending physicians. The cost differential between teaching and nonteaching hospitals may be lower when physician costs are included. This suggests that both the cost and the method of financing clinical education need to be reviewed.

An area of special concern is the method of paying teaching physicians. Teaching physicians are paid separately for their educational and patient care activities. However, these activities are frequently provided simultaneously. This has led to concerns that physicians are double billing for certain activities: for example, the physician is compensated under Medicare Part A for teaching residents and Part B for patient care service for the same patient. Although double billing is believed to be a problem, the magnitude is unknown.

It is important to recognize, however, that while the methods of financing clinical education specifically, and hospital services more generally, have changed dramatically since 1980, clinical education programs have not been forced to change significantly. Teaching hospitals earned substantial operating margins as the result of payment reform between 1980 and 1987, and the market share of teaching hospitals has increased despite the fact that charges are higher in teaching hospitals (chapter 2). The Congress has made a series of adjustments to ensure that teaching hospitals are not disproportionately affected by Medicare payment reform initiatives. Medicaid programs in several states have similarly analyzed and adjusted their payment schemes to ensure that teaching hospitals are not adversely affected by payment reform.

However, the continued financing of clinical education programs through such reimbursement adjustments and the financial strength of teaching hospitals are not assured. A recent federal advisory council has questioned whether or not the Medicare program should continue to support clinical education (Aiken and Bays, 1984). This advisory council was simply reiterating the principles established in the original Medicare legislation: that patient revenues are not an appropriate method of financing clinical education and that a suitable alternative should be found.

Recently, conditions have been changing. Profit margins are declining for all hospitals, especially teaching hospitals. The indirect medical education adjustment has been reduced substantially. Medicaid programs are debating whether they should fund clinical education rather than programs that benefit the poor. Private insurers are wondering why they should support residency education when most analysts agree that there are already too many physicians.

Public Financing

All of the uncertainty regarding continued funding for clinical education has led to a series of debates regarding who should pay for this service. Those who propose government support of clinical education cite four reasons: (1) to maintain academic health centers, (2) to maintain residency programs, (3) to support a public good, and (4) to ensure that the appropriate quantity, specialty mix, and geographic distribution of physicians are maintained.

Academic Medical Centers

Proponents argue that academic health centers are valuable national resources that need to be preserved (Colloton, 1984). This argument is based upon the assumption that the institutions, not just the services, should be preserved. Academic health centers are said to be at a significant financial disadvantage in a price sensitive environment because of the added costs associated with training programs.

Data presented in chapters 1 and 2 do not support the concern that teaching hospitals are in financial jeopardy. Occupancy rates in teaching hospitals are relatively stable, and market share is growing compared to community hospitals. With Medicare payment rates tied in part to the ratio of residents per bed, large teaching hospitals have done especially well financially. As a consequence, congressional policy makers have begun to question the necessity of continuing to level the playing field for these hospitals and to question whether federal funds should be used to maintain the current set of institutions (Anderson and Lave, 1985). There is no special reason that the current number of hospitals should be maintained or that each institution should continue its current level of clinical education. The decision to fortify the academic health center by leveling the playing field has become an indirect way of covering the cost of services that society has been unwilling to fund explicitly.

Residency Programs

A second reason frequently presented for financing residency training is the need to maintain a postgraduate slot for each medical school graduate. Since the 1930s, there have consistently been more residency positions available than graduates to fill them (table 4-2). However, since 1970 the ratio of graduates to slots has declined steadily. This has caused concern within the medical community over whether there will be enough positions available to train all graduates of medical schools. Some contend that because one year of residency training is required for licensure, a slot must be guaranteed for each physician seeking one.

Given the current aggregate supply of physicians, it may no longer be necessary to ensure each graduate a slot. If fewer positions were available, the market would determine who receives graduate medical training. In theory, the most qualified graduates would get positions and fewer of the less qualified would receive training, possibly raising the overall quality of medical care.

In addition, medicine is the only profession that receives public funds to pay for the cost of advanced training required for licensure. Public funds are not used to support the training of architects, who are required to complete a three-year apprenticeship prior to licensure eligibility. It is unclear what differentiates physicians from other professionals in their need for public support of postgraduate training. Nor do we guarantee everyone wishing to enter medical school a place by using public funds to insure that the supply matches the demand for training. It is unclear why they should be granted a position after they finish medical school.

Public Good

A third argument, the view held by many within the medical profession, is that medical education should continue to be funded through patient care revenues because it is a public good (Nash, 1987). Although medical education benefits the public to the extent that it trains qualified physicians to meet our nation's health care needs, it does not meet the standard economic definition of a public good. A public good is a commodity or a service supplied by the government that benefits all citizens. It must be provided collectively to consumers or not at all. Moreover, if the good is provided to some consumers there is no additional cost of providing it to all consumers. The traditional example of a public good is a coastal lighthouse. The lighthouse benefits everyone and yet it does not cost any more to operate if there are zero or a million users. It is usually a characteristic of such goods that it is difficult to exclude consumers from the consumption of these goods even if they have not paid for them. These characteristics do not apply to residency education.

A second argument against considering graduate medical education a public good is undergraduate medical education. If it is appropriate to fund graduate medical education as a public good, then we should be funding undergraduate medical training as well. Undergraduate medical education provides general medical training, whereas graduate medical education frequently provides highly specialized training often in specialties where supply already exceeds the perceived national need. However, medical education at the undergraduate level has not been treated as a public good. Although federal and state governments have at various times supported undergraduate medical education through scholarship funds, direct appropriations, and block grants, this support was not provided under the argument that medical education is a public good. These funds, which have been curtailed in recent years, were provided to address specific perceived shortages in overall supply or in geographic or specialty maldistributions. In summary, graduate medical education may be a service that benefits the public but it is not, strictly speaking, a public good.

Public Financing for Selected Programs

Each of the above arguments have been used to advocate the financing of graduate medical education. Given our position that these reasons for public sponsorship of clinical education programs are not justified, it is appropriate to reconsider the basis for public funding of clinical education, to ask what the role of the private sector should be, to determine whether the government has a legitimate role in financing clinical education and, if so, to ask what that role should be.

If, as a nation, we believe that access to a basic package of medical care should be provided, then it may be incumbent on the government to ensure that these services are available. To fulfill this requirement, physicians and other health professionals need to be trained in the specialties that will meet our national health care needs and need to be encouraged to practice in medically underserved areas. It is unclear why all residency programs should be supported, however.

Education programs do not add significantly to the total cost when both physician and hospital costs are considered together. Since most studies show that we have an adequate supply of physicians, and indeed a projected oversupply, public funds may not be needed to support the training of all physicians. To the extent that the market is capable of supporting medical education, financing should be derived from patient care revenues.

In the event that the market fails to provide enough support to produce the number of physicians with specified qualifications to meet the nation's health care needs, public funds should be used to finance clinical education programs to ensure that the appropriate quantity, quality, specialty mix, and geographic distribution are maintained (Kindig, 1982). This may require special funding for specialties such as geriatrics or creating financial incentives for physicians to locate in medically underserved areas. Because it is unlikely that the market will provide an ideal distribution, public involvement may be required in order to influence specialty and geographic distribution as a means of ensuring access to a basic level of medical care across the nation.

Numerous methods of federal financing of graduate medical education have been proposed recently, all of them designed with the aim of influencing the distribution of physicians. Each of these proposals has included the continuation of public support for the direct costs of graduate medical education. Some proposals would limit the number of years of financing for graduate medical education. One calls for funding the first three years of residency training, while another would provide funding for residents up to the first point of eligibility for board certification (Heyssel, 1984). Other proposals have called for the elimination of funding for foreign-born FMGs or for all FMGs (Petersdorf, 1985). Another proposal has attempted to combine federal financing and manpower policy to address the need to redistribute the supply of physicians across specialties. Under this proposal, federal payments for direct education costs would be differentiated across specialties, with areas of need receiving higher payments than areas of oversupply (Anderson and Rapoza, 1985).

Others have suggested that financing of graduate medical education is not a federal responsibility but should be shouldered by the private sector entirely. These proposals typically focus on identifying who receives the benefit of graduate medical education and suggest that the beneficiary finance the cost. Some believe that the resident is the primary beneficiary, while others believe it is the attending physician, the hospital, or the patients. In some scenarios, the cost is shared among multiple beneficiaries.

The Need for Change

Our recommendation for developing a new method of financing clinical education is based on several assumptions. First, the current system for financing graduate medical education is not broken; teaching hospitals are still training physicians and being paid for it, whether explicitly or implicitly. Although hospitals may be able to continue cross-subsidizing clinical education with patient care revenues in the short run, the competitive pricing of hospital services may reduce the extent that they are able to do so over a long period. In addition, explicit payments for graduate medical education have been reduced and are likely to decline further. Consequently, it may be risky to depend on the current system of financing to sustain clinical training in the future.

Second, if current funding mechanisms change, the structure, breadth, and quantity of educational programs may also change. Since adequately trained health professionals are needed to provide medical care, one of the objectives of our proposed financing system is to anticipate the future so a new financing scheme is operational before changes in the health care environment adversely affect the supply of medical personnel.

Third, even if the financing system remains unchanged, a new method of funding graduate medical education is needed, because the current payment system is unresponsive to certain public policy objectives, such as a better distribution of physicians. Finally, the current system of financing is not based on the cost of providing the service and on who receives the benefit.

Objectives

One objective of our proposal is to ensure that an appropriate balance is established and maintained regarding the quantity and distribution of trained physicians across both specialties and geographic areas. According to most studies, the market does not distribute physicians geographically or across specialties according to the health care needs of the nation as a whole. To the extent that physicians in specific specialties are needed to ensure access to appropriate care, the federal government may have to intervene in the market by creating incentives for physicians to choose certain specialties. The same responsibility holds for influencing the geographic choices of physicians emerging from their training.

The second objective of this proposal is to pay the full cost of services rendered. Residents and interns provide significant patient care services. Indeed, studies show that residents in their first year of graduate training spend 50–75 percent of their time providing patient care (Feldman, 1976; Yoder, 1977). We believe that residents should be compensated for the services they provide and that the current system should be changed to allow their services to be billed for on a fee-for-service basis.

There has been an ongoing debate for decades concerning the status of residents. Are they students or employees? The prevailing position in the medical community is that residents are students whose primary role is to learn rather than provide services during the training period (New York State Commission, 1986). This view presents residents as students engaged in apprentice-style on-the-job training. Residents, on the other hand, tend to define themselves as employees and emphasize their contribution to patient care. Some residents have sought recognition as junior faculty members at associated medical schools, while others have conducted vigorous job actions.

As the health care system evolves, it will be increasingly important to resolve the issue of the resident's status (Lee and Hadley, 1985). If we define residents as students, it would be appropriate to finance graduate medical education via tuition payments or private funds, such as scholarships or grants. If we choose instead to treat residents as employees participating in an apprenticeship, graduate medical education would be financed by paying directly for their services. In fact, residents perform a dual role; they are both students and employees. However, we believe that, on balance they act more as apprentices, providing more patient care services than receiving training and therefore should be paid for their services.

The key characteristic of apprenticeship training is that it is general and therefore transferable (Becker and Steinwald, 1981). The hospital or medical care site sponsoring a training program is making an investment in these physicians and receiving some benefit at the time of training. But what about the future? The sponsor does not stand to gain in the long term from its investment, because the fully trained physician can go into the market and command a higher wage rate based on his or her new skill level. Based on economic theory, a rational firm in a competitive labor market would not be willing to bear the cost of the training. Individuals receiving the training should be willing to bear the cost, since their future earning potential increases with general training. Therefore, the trainee, not the firm, typically pays for this training by accepting lower wages during the period of training. This argues in favor of lower wages for the resident during the course of the residency in return for increased future earning potential. As a group, physicians are well paid relative to other professionals. Indeed, studies indicate that physicians earn a significant return on their training investment once they are in practice (Burstein and Cromwell, 1985; Feldman, 1976; Lee, 1984).

A third objective of this proposal is to construct a financing mechanism that will allow those who benefit from graduate medical education to bear the cost of training. There are four primary beneficiaries of graduate medical education: (1) trainees, (2) physicians, (3) the training site, and (4) patients. Residents increase their future earning potential through additional training. Residents support fully trained physicians by providing medical care to their patients, thus allowing the supervising physician to treat more patients and freeing them of their on-call responsibilities for hospitalized patients. The training site also benefits, since residents perform a significant amount of the medical care for hospitalized patients and substitute for hospital personnel. Medical education may also add to the prestige of an institution thus enhancing the hospital's market share. Finally, the patient benefits directly through the medical services provided by the resident.

Our Proposal for Financing Clinical Education

Step One

Eliminate third-party payments for direct and indirect costs of all clinical education training programs. The current system finances the direct costs for all residency and some fellowship training plus salary support for residency supervision and administration. These funds are generated explicitly via Medicare Part A and implicitly by other third-party payors through higher reimbursement levels, which are set, in part, to cover the costs of clinical education. Our proposal would eliminate all third-party implicit and explicit subsidies for the direct costs of clinical education, making all payors equal with respect to payments for clinical education.

The proposal also calls for eliminating funding of the indirect costs of graduate medical education. The Medicare allocation for indirect medical education has been a proxy for a variety of factors contributing to the greater cost of patient care in teaching hospitals. Many of these factors are unrelated to teaching, such as severity of illness. In chapter 7, we discussed proposed adjustments to the prospective payment system which would pay explicitly for these factors. Refining PPS in this manner would reduce estimates of the indirect costs attributable to medical education to 4 or 5 percent per resident for every ten hospital beds (see chapters 1 and 4).

When physician payments are combined with the cost of hospitals, the incremental cost of clinical education is further reduced to less than 2 percent for each resident per ten beds (chapter 4). Under the proposed plan, the cost of training physicians would be the responsibility of the hospital, the faculty practice plan, or the outpatient setting sponsoring the educational program. Since this organization benefits from the presence of graduate medical education, it shares in the cost.

A possible outcome of requiring hospitals to sponsor a portion of the cost of training is that some hospitals may no longer be willing to provide educational programs. This could pose problems for delivery of care to the poor and uninsured. As we discussed in chapter 6, a disproportionate share of medical care for this group is provided by public teaching hospitals. If the number of residents was reduced or educational programs were eliminated in these hospitals, access to care for the medically indigent could be adversely affected. This problem is discussed in chapter 10.

Step Two

Allow all personal and identifiable services performed by residents in an accredited program to be billed for on a fee-for-service basis. The billing for residents' services would be the responsibility of the hospital, faculty practice plan, or ambulatory group sponsoring the accredited residency program. Residents' salaries would be paid through the revenue generated by those fees. Any revenues generated in excess of the predetermined salary and fringe benefits would be retained by the sponsor. Similarly, any revenue shortfalls would be covered by the sponsor. Thus, residents' incomes are not dependent explicitly on the revenues generated through their patient care.

This plan can address the need to more closely connect developing patterns in delivery of care and in training location. As delivery patterns of medical care change, the site and content of training need to change as well. Current reimbursement policies for graduate medical education pay for training in the hospital but often do not pay for education conducted in alternative delivery sites, such as ambulatory centers or HMOs. This is one reason that alternative delivery sites have not participated very extensively in training. The proposed financing scheme would allow billing for residents' services regardless of site, thus eliminating the financial disadvantage to using nonhospital locations for training. If this change is not enough to persuade nonhospital sites to participate in training physicians, explicit incentives can be established to encourage these sites to become involved.

One mechanism to consider is a grants program funded by the federal government (see step four).

In an era of budget deficits and rising health care costs, this financing system can be made budget neutral. This proposal shifts payment for direct medical education costs from the hospital to the physician component—or in the federal government's case, from Medicare Part A to Part B. As Part A expenses decline, Part B costs increase. By adjusting Part B payment rates, the system can be made budget neutral. It would have the additional benefit of reducing or eliminating the possibility of double billing by attending physicians.

This proposal would not have a major financial impact on most academic medical centers. When hospital and physician costs are combined and all of the differences in cost of living, case mix, and care for low-income patients are taken into account, teaching programs do not increase costs substantially (chapter 4). In most institutions, the incremental hospital and physician costs associated with residency programs are less than five percent. Given the possibility of higher charges and increased market share associated with the imprimatur of a teaching program, the investment is probably warranted simply on financial terms. The proposals would, however, shift resources from physicians to hospitals.

Billing on a fee-for-service basis creates a more equitable system in which all third-party payors pay their proportionate share of direct costs of graduate medical education. In addition, training programs become self-supporting, since payors are paying for residents' services. Further, teaching hospitals in a price-sensitive environment may benefit because, with these costs financed separately, hospitals can recalculate patient care charges, removing residency salary costs and thus reducing hospital costs and charges.

Billing for residents' services on a fee-for-service basis requires changing state laws to allow services performed by first-year residents to be reimbursed. Currently, physicians cannot bill for their professional services until they are licensed, which is generally contingent on passing Part 3 of the National Medical Boards and completing one year of postgraduate training (requirements vary by state).

There is some concern, however, that physicians coming directly out of medical school (interns) are not equipped to act as the primary physician in providing patient care. Some question the ability of interns to provide the services required and the extent to which their work can be unsupervised. If it is determined that interns are not prepared to act independently enough to provide separate and identifiable services, we would recommend incorporating the internship into the domain of the medical school. Medical schooling would be lengthened from four to five years and would prepare graduates to actually practice medicine under supervision.

This system creates new incentives, which need to be monitored. First, there is a potential for overworking residents. The more patients treated, the more professional fees generated. This means programs may require residents to work longer hours or to look for the most efficient residents. At the same time, most productivity studies suggest that residents' output declines after a certain number of hours.

Second, certain types of residency programs will be more appealing than others. Procedure-oriented specialties will have greater financial incentives to train residents than cognitive specialties, because prevailing Medicare rates are higher. Thus a first-year resident in neurosurgery is more valuable financially to a hospital or a practice plan than a pediatrics resident because of the significant reimbursement differential. This introduces the larger issue of physician payment reform. Finally, this financing plan creates competition between the resident and the attending physician for professional fees.

Step Three

Establish specific requirements for the supervision of residents. Residents learn by doing; consequently, their work will continue to need supervision. Because this financing system alters incentives, it will be important to monitor the quality of the educational programs and the quality of care provided. One of the issues this raises is where the locus of control is best placed, in the hospital or in the medical school. A recurring debate within the medical community is whether medical schools should be responsible for the quality of graduate medical education programs (New York State Commission, 1986). It is believed that medical school affiliation would provide safeguards for quality, because the medical school would not want to be associated with a poor quality residency program.

Under our plan, all residency programs, to be accredited, would be required to affiliate with a medical school. If the training program was of poor quality to begin with, it would have difficulty affiliating. If, on the other hand, the medical school was already affiliated with a program, it would have an incentive to maintain quality and thus would be likely to participate in clinical training to ensure quality. In this way, residency education would be a continuation of the educational process.

Step Four

Government intervention is needed to fulfill specialty and geographic requirements. Geographic and specialty distribution of physicians should be monitored. Past federal and state attempts to address geographic and specialty maldistribution have not been broad based, systematic, or effective (chapter 4). Nor has the market been successful in producing the supply of physicians required by specialty or locale.

If the market is not producing the quantity, quality, and specialty and geographic mix of physicians to meet the minimal standards of access to care as defined by federal manpower policy, then the federal government should intervene. The interim measure to address this issue is to develop a federal grant program to support specific residency programs. The grants would be targeted to areas of specialty need and would be funded only when a shortage of these specialists was projected. Staffing needs would have to be projected for ten to fifteen years in the future because of the length of the training pipeline.

The preferred solution to controlling specialty and geographic distribution in the long term is to reform the physician payment system by differentially paying physicians geographically and by specialty. This requires the development of an alternative physician payment system. If, for example, more geriatricians are needed and we have an oversupply of neurosurgeons, the federal government might alter physician reimbursement levels for the Medicare program, making the differential large enough to attract medical school graduates to these programs. The same principle could be applied to fulfilling geographic staffing needs.

chapter 9 | Biomedical Research

Very little is known about the extent or the costs of the biomedical research and technology development conducted in hospitals. Revenues from patient care services have been available to subsidize research projects, and thus hospitals have had no serious economic incentive to identify their costs. Third-party payors have been paying for this research implicitly through higher patient care charges or costs.

As the ability to cross-subsidize services diminishes, the willingness of the hospital to subsidize biomedical research may change. The method of financing clinical education could have a significant influence on what types of research are conducted, where research is conducted, and the rate of diffusion of new technologies. For these reasons, it is important to examine a number of policy issues related to these services. Specifically, we should determine the extent and total cost of biomedical research and technological development occurring in hospitals. The next step is to develop alternative sources of funding. Finally, it is necessary to determine how resources are allocated within the academic medical center and to suggest modifications to the current system.

Step One

Collect additional data on the extent and cost of clinical research. The extent and cost of biomedical research and technology development has never been adequately investigated. Several important questions remain unanswered. First, what types of clinical research are conducted in hospitals? Hospital administrators generally have data on externally sponsored research projects, such as grants from NIH, and major internal projects, such as organ transplant programs. However, most hospital administrators do not have data on the extent or

187

cost of unsponsored projects, such as the additional time spent by surgeons developing new procedures in the operating room. As a result, the full extent of clinical research is frequently unknown at the hospital level and is most certainly unknown at the national level.

Another question is, where is research and technology development being conducted? Funding data showed that sponsored research is conducted in a relatively small number of academic medical centers (chapter 5). Although the same level of concentration may exist for unsponsored biomedical research and technology developments, it is possible that unsponsored research is more broadly based, since physicians trained in research environments practice in other types of hospitals.

The third question is, what are the costs associated with biomedical research and technology development? Once projects are identified, it is necessary to determine the cost to each project. As discussed in chapter 5, few studies have attempted to quantify the cost of biomedical research or technology development. A methodology similar to that used to identify the cost of clinical education (chapter 4) may be the best place to begin to determine the cost of clinical research.

Step Two

Publicly fund clinical research; give funds directly to the hospital, and base the aggregate level of funding on national priorities. Hospital-based clinical research supported through internal funds was relatively easy to finance under the cost-based and charge-based reimbursement systems. As reforms in the hospital financing system continue, it may be necessary to change the method of financing biomedical research and technology development. Because research lends hospitals a comparative advantage by allowing them to differentiate their product, they are likely to continue using some of their own resources to finance clinical research. However, one would expect to see the extent of internally sponsored clinical research decrease as the ability to cross-subsidize diminishes. Policy makers need to review current methods of financing these services and ensure that changes in hospital reimbursement do not eliminate internally sponsored research.

Unlike clinical education, biomedical research and technology development are public goods in the traditional welfare economics sense, meaning that they benefit everyone and it is impossible to exclude anyone from the benefit. During the past fifty years, the federal government has taken the lead in financing biomedical research. The research conducted in clinical settings is important to the advancement of medical care and often leads to real innovation in clinical practice. Results from this research are distributed through publication in peer-reviewed journals. As a result, these clinical innovations are incorporated more broadly by practitioners until they become the standard of medical practice. Benefits from these advances accrue to the public, collectively. No single individual or corporation captures these benefits to the exclusion of others.

Much of the clinical research traditionally funded by hospitals using internal funds is a public good. Therefore, it is appropriate for the federal government to provide some level of funding for these activities to ensure that these projects are continued. An option is to use federal grants to support this research. The grant would be made directly to the hospital to continue its program of technology development and clinical research. A prototype for this type of financing exists in the biomedical research support grants (BRSG) from NIH. Institutions with at least three NIH grants of $200,000 or more are eligible to apply for these grants. Awards are made annually in one lump sum to the institutions free of requirements on how the funds are distributed. Disbursement of these funds is based on institutional priorities. In general, BRSG awards are made to universities and not to hospitals.

We propose that the method of financing clinical research be changed and incorporated into the current system of federal funding through the NIH extramural grants program. To make this possible, NIH may need to broaden the definition of appropriate research activity to incorporate more applied biomedical research and technology development. Hospitals would apply to NIH under the current grant-making system for extramural research funding. This would require hospitals to define the programs they currently sponsor through cross-subsidies, particularly internally sponsored clinical research, and to determine the costs of those projects. Applications for these projects would be judged on a competitive basis under the peer review process. Hospitals would then receive grants based on merit. Renewal of the grant would be based on performance. "If after a period of three years or so, the institution cannot justify the payment on the basis of performance, they lose it and will have to cut costs to remain competitive on price" (Heyssel, 1984, p. 114).

This proposal does not suggest that it is necessary for the federal government to fund everything hospitals request or even to fund all of the projects that hospitals have funded in the past. It should be left to the political process to determine general research priorities. Hospitals that wish to continue to fund research and technology development but do not receive direct funding would be free to continue at their own expense.

This change in financing would allow the acknowledgement of the value and importance of clinical research and to finance a portion of it explicitly. In the event that hospitals fund fewer of these projects through cross-subsidies in the future, thus hindering progress in biomedical research and technology development, a system would already be operational to fund projects that contribute to the general welfare of the nation.

Step Three

Require sponsors of clinical research to pay the full cost of conducting the research. It is unlikely that the federal government and private corporations have paid the full cost of clinical research in the past (chapter 5). When these underfunded projects are hospital based, the hospital frequently absorbs the uncovered costs. Hospitals have not been very concerned about this expense, since the higher costs are incorporated into the hospital's cost base and are ultimately paid by patients.

Requiring the government to ensure that the full cost is covered may result in fewer research grants being awarded. If total funding remains constant but sponsored grants are funded at their actual cost, the number of grants awarded will decline. This is ultimately a matter of federal budget priorities.

The issue is more serious for private industry sponsors. In the United States, hospitals and medical schools generally require pharmaceutical firms and equipment manufacturers conducting clinical trials to pay for the cost of the clinical trial. In many foreign countries, however, the cost of the clinical trial is paid by the government as part of the national health service. This creates an economic incentive for U.S. manufacturers to conduct clinical trials outside the United States. Recently, the Food and Drug Administration has become increasingly willing to accept clinical trials conducted in foreign countries. If the cost of conducting research projects increases, the exodus would also probably increase. If this process continues, it is possible that the United States will lose scientists to foreign countries, where an increasing number of clinical trials will be conducted.

Step Four

Academic medical centers should review their allocation of overhead (indirect costs) between the hospital and university to determine whether some of the revenues should be transferred to hospitals. In most academic medical centers, reimbursement for overhead cost is captured by the medical school. Medical schools and universities receiving NIH and other grants should be encouraged to ensure that hospitals receive a fair share of the overhead costs paid by the grant.

chapter 10 | Uncompensated Care

Nearly 37 million nonelderly Americans were without any health insurance at some point during 1986 (U.S. Bureau of the Census, 1986). As a group, these uninsured persons tend to receive fewer medical services and possibly less appropriate treatment than the insured population (Freeman et al., 1987). For uninsured persons, access to hospital care frequently depends upon the charitable mission of individual hospitals and the ability of each hospital to cover uncompensated care through philanthropic support, public appropriations, and cross-subsidization.

Chapter 6 discusses in some detail the problems of the uninsured and the related problems of hospitals that provide uncompensated care. It concludes with a comparison of policy options that have been proposed or enacted to alleviate the problems faced by the uninsured and the hospitals that treat them. In this chapter we present our own proposal.

Evaluating the Alternatives

As discussed in chapter 6, most policy options can be grouped into three categories. The first strategy prevents hospitals from "dumping" or from failing to admit medically unstable patients. The second approach subsidizes hospitals that provide a large amount of uncompensated care. The third strategy is to reduce the number of uninsured people.

Trying to prevent hospitals from dumping patients is relatively difficult to enforce. Individual cases must be reviewed to determine if a particular patient was treated inappropriately. This process is generally time consuming and can be extremely expensive if many cases are investigated. Of greater concern, however, is that it does not attempt to solve the larger problem: it does little to discourage hospitals from dumping patients, and does even less to provide uninsured people appropriate medical treatment. Antidumping laws, therefore, may well be effective for identifying isolated incidents of inappropriate transfers, but it is not a long term solution to the problems of the uninsured and underinsured.

The second approach, one that has been preferred historically, is to subsidize hospitals that provide charity care. A number of financing schemes have been used to compensate these hospitals. State and local governments typically appropriate funds to public hospitals to support care for the poor and uninsured. Since 1981, Medicare and Medicaid laws have been amended to allow an increase in payment rates to hospitals that provide care for the poor. Some states have established programs to distribute funds to hospitals that provide a disproportionate share of uncompensated care, including indigent care pools and rate-setting programs. All of these approaches are discussed in greater detail in chapter 6.

The approach of making payments to providers rather than making health insurance more widely available has several advantages. It offers some protection to hospitals that provide a disproportionate amount of charity care and, at least indirectly, makes it possible for the uninsured to receive essential hospital services. This strategy subsidizes the cost of caring for the uninsured without increasing the number of people who are covered under entitlement programs. Further, it eliminates financial advantages for hospitals that do not provide uncompensated care. Finally, in contrast to new insurance programs, it does not create incentives for insured people to give up privately obtained health insurance or cut back on their own expenditures (Wilensky, 1986).

However, the approach of making payments to hospitals rather than extending health insurance protection to uninsured individuals raises a number of serious issues. The most fundamental concern is that this approach will probably not alleviate access problems for sick, uninsured people. Payments to hospitals for care for the poor rarely cover the full cost of treating uninsured patients. Hospitals therefore have some incentive to discriminate against these patients in favor of fully covered individuals. Even in the unlikely event that hospitals were fully reimbursed for charity care, uninsured individuals may not necessarily behave as if they were entitled to treatment for non-emergency medical conditions. Without this real sense of entitlement to health care, the uninsured may delay or avoid medically necessary treatment. This has been shown to have a deleterious effect on their health status.

Appropriateness of care is a second major problem. If hospitals, but not other health care providers, are reimbursed for treating charity care patients, a perverse incentive is created for patients to use hospital services, although less expensive and perhaps more appropriate services are available. The approach of assisting hospitals does not create an incentive for the uninsured to seek out the most efficient providers of care. Ultimately, this may make it more difficult for payors to control costs (Wilensky, 1986).

A third area of concern with an approach that compensates providers involves the role of the public hospital. As the demand for public hospital services increases, it is questionable whether or not the magnitude of resources distributed to public providers would be sufficient to cover costs. Without sufficient funding, there is a strong possibility that the quality of services provided in public hospitals would deteriorate. The concentration of a large proportion of the poor in underfunded public hospitals would be likely to exacerbate any tendency toward a two-tiered health care system. Finally, even if public hospitals were fully funded and were considered the primary provider for all uninsured persons, it would invariably be difficult because of time and travel costs for some people to have access to the nearest public hospital.

The third strategy is to decrease the number of uninsured persons by making health insurance coverage more widely available. The main advantages of this approach include increased access to the health care delivery system and improvements in health status. Because insurance coverage has been associated with increases in service utilization, this approach is likely to have a more positive effect on health status than either alternative strategy (chapter 6). It would provide newly covered individuals with some financial protection against the high cost of medical care services. It could lead to more efficient and appropriate use of health care services, while reducing the burden on public hospitals, and it could decrease the amount of uncompensated care provided by all hospitals. Ultimately, the expansion of health insurance coverage would benefit those hospitals that provide a disproportionate share of services to the uninsured.

The major disadvantage of expanding eligibility for health insurance care is that it would be more costly than the other approaches. As we discussed in chapter 6, insurance tends to improve access and increase utilization of health care services. By increasing the number of people with access to the health care delivery system, total expenditures for health care would inevitably increase. If, however, insurance packages would allow people to receive medical treatment in the most appropriate setting (primary care in the physician's office or clinic rather than in emergency rooms), then cost increases may be minimized (Wilensky, 1986).

Selecting a Strategy

In a period of constrained financial resources, the question is whether resources should be allocated to hospitals that treat the uninsured or to the uninsured themselves. Reviewing the advantages and disadvantages of the different strategies suggests that available resources should be spent on the uninsured and not the hospitals. The challenge is to design a system that would extend coverage and be implemented at minimal cost.

Some believe that the public sector should assume full responsibility for conferring coverage to the uninsured by creating a national health insurance plan. Despite the conceptual appeal of a national health insurance program, there is substantial resistance to such proposals. One concern is the cost. Because the Congress is engaged in efforts to control federal spending, national health insurance has not been actively considered in years. Moreover, many believe that existing insurance mechanisms are working well, that the private sector, complemented by Medicare, Medicaid, and other public programs, is fully capable of covering the vast majority of people, and that a system that seems to work well enough for nearly 200 million Americans should not be dismantled.

In recent years, there has been renewed interest in expanding the role of the private sector to extend coverage to portions of the uninsured population. Because close to two-thirds of the uninsured population are in the labor force or are dependents of workers, the Congress has considered numerous proposals that would require employers to extend coverage to employees, including the newly unemployed and their dependents.

While mandated coverage proposals appeal to a principle of fairness, this approach is likely to result in undesired employment and wage effects (Monheit, Hagan, and Berk, 1985). If all employers were required to offer health insurance to all employees, the fixed costs per employee could increase to a point where both employment and wages would be reduced (U.S. Congress, Congressional Budget Office, 1987). The most deleterious effects are likely to be experienced by low-wage workers, who represent a large portion of the uninsured work force.

Moreover, without some mechanism for insuring the unemployed, mandated coverage could leave as many as fifteen million Americans still without health insurance.

Another approach that has received some attention would allow people without health insurance to buy into Medicaid programs. Typically, Medicaid buy-in proposals involve a copayment from individuals, which would increase with the individual's income. Such proposals appear to provide a relatively simple method of extending coverage by building onto existing state programs, rather than creating new ones. However, the Medicaid buy-in approach has several limitations. For example, it is unlikely that low-income uninsured people will be able to afford out-of-pocket payments to buy Medicaid coverage. Without a subsidy, some low-income individuals who need health coverage would therefore not benefit from the new program. A second issue is cost. Assuming that individual payments were insufficient to cover the additional costs incurred by the expanded Medicaid program, it is not clear how the new programs would be financed. A third problem could be low participation rates, if the stigma of coverage under Medicaid prevents some uninsured people from signing up for the new program.

Our Proposal for Covering the Uninsured

Step One

Treat all employer contributions to health insurance as taxable employee income. Since the 1940s, the tax code has been used to subsidize the cost of employer-based health insurance. During World War II, fringe benefits were excluded from wage controls in order to allow real wages to rise. In 1954, employer contributions to health coverage were deemed to be nontaxable.

There are two distinct problems with the current tax policy (Enthoven, 1980). First, the value of the exemption increases with income, while the cost of insurance does not increase. For example, in 1983, the exemption was worth $622 for families with incomes between $50,000 and $100,000, but only $83 to families with incomes between $10,000 and $15,000 (Enthoven, 1985). With changes in rates enacted in the 1986 Tax Reform Act, the disparity in tax benefits may not be quite as wide but would persist, nonetheless. Second, the current tax benefit excludes over twenty million people who do not have access to employer-sponsored health coverage. Even with the new provision that allows the self-employed to deduct 25 percent of premium costs, millions of uninsured Americans are unable to benefit from the tax deduction in the revised tax law. The tax code as currently written subsidizes the cost of insurance but fails to spread the subsidy evenly across all Americans.

Eliminating the tax deduction for health insurance would provide additional tax revenues of 34.3 billion in 1989 (U.S. Congress, Congressional Budget Office, 1987). Of course, there are other methods of raising tax revenues, such as a change in the marginal tax rates or an income tax surcharge. Depending on how these taxes are enacted, they could be more or less progressive than the elimination of the tax deduction for health insurance. We chose to eliminate the tax deduction for employer contributions to health insurance to keep all of the initiatives within the health sphere.

Step Two

Use new revenues to provide a refundable tax credit that will be dedicated exclusively to the purchase of health insurance. Every individual (and family) would be eligible to receive a tax credit. The value of the credit would be larger for two-person and multiperson families. Our proposal involves a dedicated, refundable tax credit that would be available to all potential purchasers of health insurance (excluding only Medicare and Medicaid beneficiaries), not simply those with employer-paid health insurance and those who are self-employed. In contrast to the existing system of tax exclusions, this tax credit is a more progressive approach. The dollar value of the credit does not increase with income; it is the same for everyone, regardless of income.

To calculate the value of the credit, we began with an estimate of the cost to the federal government of excluding employer contributions from taxable employee income. In fiscal year 1989, when the recent reform of the tax code is fully implemented, the full cost of excluding health insurance premiums from taxation is estimated to be $34.3 billion (U.S. Congress, Congressional Budget Office, 1987). We divided $34.3 billion among individual, two-person, and multiperson families, giving a larger tax credit to two-person families and an even larger credit to multiperson families. We increased the value of the credit according to family size to account for the relative difference in the cost of insurance. We reviewed price differentials in several

plans for individual, two-person, and multiperson families and assumed a purchasing price in 1989 for a minimum health insurance
package of $1,000, $2,000, and $2,600, respectively. Based upon the
number of people in each category, we estimate a 1989 refundable tax
credit of $222 for individuals, $444 for two-person families, and $577
for multiperson families.[1]

This approach has several advantages. First, because the tax
credit would reduce the price of insurance for all persons and because
it can be used only to purchase health insurance, it should stimulate
the demand for health coverage among those who are currently uninsured. Second, because the tax credit would simply redistribute for-
gone tax revenues, it is designed to be budget neutral. Third, because
the credit is refundable, those who do not owe taxes would still benefit
directly. In contrast to tax credits that are of value only to those who
pay taxes, a refundable tax credit is a subsidy available to everyone
providing they file a tax form. Fourth, the tax credit would not discourage employees from purchasing health insurance from their employers, given the price advantages associated with group rates. We
would expect that employees would still prefer employer-based insurance and that employers would be willing to incur the administrative
expense of providing group insurance. We believe this approach is
unlikely to threaten existing mechanisms for purchasing health insurance, which is a considerable advantage given that 180 million people
are currently covered by employer-provided benefits.

Step Three

Subsidize the cost of insurance for persons who are poor and near
poor. Even with the refundable tax credit, many poor and near poor
uninsured persons would be unable to afford even the least expensive
insurance policy. By itself, a tax credit may be insufficient as an incentive to induce many low-income consumers to purchase insurance.
There is therefore concern that a tax credit for health insurance would

---

1. To determine the value of the tax credit, we used the 1985 Current Population
Survey to break out the number of individual, two-person, and multiperson family units
that would be eligible to receive a tax credit; they were 21.7 million, 19.0 million, and
36.4 million, respectively (persons age sixty-five or older, were excluded). The tax credit
increases by the ratio of relative prices for two-person and multiperson families. We
then divided the estimate cost of the tax exclusion for employer-based premiums for
fiscal year 1989 by the number of family units, adjusting for the relative price difference:

$34.3 billion $= 21.7X + 19.0(2.0)X + 36.4(2.6)X.$ (X = $222 for individuals.)

leave many uninsured persons in the same position that they are in today. Because large numbers of poor and near poor uninsured persons would not have enough income to buy their own insurance without either adjustments in price or some sort of subsidy, our proposal would subsidize the cost of insurance, varying the subsidy by income.

To calculate the value of the subsidy, we started with family income and made a series of decisions about a person's ability to pay. Our objective was to derive a relatively simple formula that would allow individuals to contribute a reasonable amount based upon income. In the formula that we chose, we decided that maximum family liability for health insurance, including the tax credit, should be no more than 15 percent of adjusted income. To guarantee that very low income people would not have to pay anything, we deducted $3,000 from family income. If the tax credit was less than 15 percent of the family income, the individual would pay the difference between the tax credit and the maximum liability, and the government would fund the difference. If the tax credit exceeded 15 percent of adjusted income, the individual or family would not be expected to make additional payments. Individuals not eligible for the subsidy would pay the full cost of the insurance above the value of the tax credit. This takes into account the fact that some uninsured persons have sufficient resources to be able to pay for their own health insurance.

The result of our subsidy program is that out-of-pocket expenditures increase with family income, and government subsidies are targeted to help those who might otherwise be unable to afford health insurance. The following example of a two-person family with an income of $6,500 illustrates how the formula works. First, we deduct $3,000 from family income. We multiply the adjusted income $3,500 by 15 percent to get a maximum subscriber liability of $525. Because the family has not exceeded the maximum out-of-pocket expenditures by contributing the $444 refundable tax credit, it would pay an additional $81 per year. The government would pay the full difference ($1,475) between the cost of insurance ($2,000) and the maximum subscriber liability ($525), including the $444 tax credit.

Special provisions would be necessary to prevent states from dismantling their Medicaid programs. For persons living above the poverty level who are eligible for the subsidy, the federal government would pay the full amount. For persons living below the poverty line who are not covered by the Medicaid program, states would be required to share the cost of the subsidy with the federal government. The increased cost to the state could be offset partially by revenues achieved by the state's taxation of employer contributions to health insurance.

The total cost of this subsidy is estimated to be a maximum of $27 billion. However, this figure is probably an overestimate, since our estimate makes the unlikely assumption that all persons eligible for the refundable credit will file a tax form, purchase health insurance, and apply for the subsidy. This assumption may be particularly questionable in the case of low-income persons who do not ordinarily file a tax form and uninsured persons who may not perceive a need for health insurance.

There are no known empirical studies that describe the extent to which a full or partial subsidy through the tax system would stimulate poor and uninsured persons to purchase health insurance. A theoretical framework would suggest that the decision to purchase insurance is based upon risk aversion, expectation of loss, price, and income, but it is not clear how well the uninsured fit into this framework. Some would argue that the transaction costs of filling out and submitting a tax form would present too great an obstacle and would deter individuals from using the tax credit and subsidy to buy insurance (Lees and Rice, 1965). We believe that a refundable tax credit, with a subsidy that increases as income decreases, would be sufficient inducement to lure eligible persons to file tax forms and to enroll in a health coverage plan.

Because the $27 billion cost estimate represents a substantial increase in public expenditures for health care, it might be useful to consider this estimate within the context of other proposals for universal health coverage. The Kennedy proposal to extend health insurance coverage through employer-mandated benefits is estimated to increase employer's costs by $27 billion but would have a minimal budgetary effect on federal, state, or local governments (Gordon, 1988). If there were no undesirable employment effects, then up to 23 of the 37 million uninsured persons would be covered by the Kennedy plan.

Step Four

Require each state to design and implement a program, to ensure that everyone has the opportunity to obtain coverage. Programs may vary by source of revenues, financing and administrative structure, and degree of private sector involvement. Our proposal would require each state to design its own plan to offer health insurance to the uninsured and also to organize the delivery of services. Many states have already adopted programs for the uninsured. We recognize that programs created as a result of this proposal should be suited to each state's economic and political environment. However, all state plans would have open enrollment and uniform eligibility criteria and minimum benefits.

All persons without health insurance for reasons of health, employment status, or income would have access to state-sponsored health insurance. Many states have implemented risk pools to cover only persons with preexisting medical conditions that preclude them from purchasing health insurance. The medically uninsurable population would be able to enroll in the state plan. Employed but uninsured persons would also have access to the state plan. Many employed and uninsured persons do not have the option of buying health insurance, because it is not offered to them or because the copayments are prohibitively expensive. Since the primary objective is to provide all uninsured persons access to health coverage, the new state plan would have no categorical exclusions.

The Congress would define the minimal benefit package to be offered by each state plan. Because federal dollars would be used to finance the plan and the coverage it buys, it is important that the federal government retain some control over the benefit package. With a defined minimum package, coverage offered to the uninsured would be consistent across states. With a federally defined benefit plan, this proposal would guard against concerns often raised with tax credit and subsidized voucher proposals: sending consumers into the marketplace without the information needed to make appropriate purchasing decisions and without assurances of coverage in minimally adequate health plan.

Maximal out-of-pocket expenditures for each state plan would be defined to assure that low-income uninsured persons were able to use their tax credit and subsidy to receive health coverage. States could choose to increase copayments for more generous plans. To be sure that the uninsured would have access to the state plan when they need it, there would be mandatory open enrollment. This is necessary, given the already low enrollment in state plans. Considerable effort would be needed to inform potential enrollees about the plan, and every effort should be made to make enrollment as easy as possible. Open enrollment would alleviate a major obstacle to access. We envision two general models: an expanded, partially subsidized, Medicaid buy-in program or a quasi-public risk pool. States could choose these or other models, as long as the program included the federally defined criteria for the minimum plan.

The approach of expanding Medicaid to include all uninsured persons could have several advantages. First, it would meet the objective of assuring that all uninsured persons have the option of buying health insurance. Second, it is likely to be a less costly way of financing coverage, since public plans tend to have lower administrative costs and may be able to use regulatory authority to negotiate lower payment rates to providers. A by-product of this approach could be that the major differences between state Medicaid programs would be eliminated. This would be true only, however, if states offer the federally defined basic insurance package to all Medicaid beneficiaries.

There are several disadvantages to placing coverage of all poor, near poor, and uninsured persons under the jurisdiction of the Medicaid program. One problem is that the unpoor uninsured may be reluctant to enroll because of the stigma of being a Medicaid beneficiary or because they do not foresee needing medical care. A second problem is the possibility that a widely expanded Medicaid program would become a substitute for private health insurance, thereby competing with the insurance industry. Third, because of relatively low Medicaid reimbursement levels in some states, there may not be sufficient providers to ensure access to health services.

States could choose instead to create a risk pool. The risk pool model has been tested in several states and is under consideration in others. The pool may be funded by general revenues, subscriber premiums, tax credits, subsidies, and whatever additional revenue sources the state deems appropriate. States could, for example, impose a tax on employers or insurers to subsidize the pool. Such a tax would be a strong incentive for employers who do not currently offer health insurance to contribute to the financing of the pool, because participation would be less costly than the tax.

An advantage to the pool option is that it would allow state governments to respond to the federal initiative to target the uninsured without the political constraints tied to the Medicaid program. A pool of all uninsured persons, not just the medically uninsurables, could achieve economies of scale, which could slow the increase in costs and reduce deficits. The major obstacle may be that the insurance industry would not support the new program. Because the federal government would define the minimum benefit package, maximum copayments, and eligibility, the insurance industry may resist participation. In the past, there has been great resistance to pools that included more than just the medically uninsurable population. States may have to offer the insurance industry some protection against economic loss.

Step Five

Eliminate Medicare and Medicaid payment adjustments to hospitals that provide a disproportionate share of uncompensated services so that, ultimately, all public subsidies can be eliminated. A final and related issue involves the interaction of this proposal with existing programs designed to support disproportionate share hospitals.

Currently, hospitals that provide a disproportionate share of services to low-income persons are eligible to receive an adjustment in their Medicare payment rate based upon the percentage of low-income patients. In fiscal year 1987, Medicare paid an estimated $500 million to disproportionate share hospitals (U.S. Congress, Congressional Budget Office, unpublished estimate). If our proposal was fully implemented, payments to providers would be duplicative and should therefore be discontinued. This would be especially true if appropriate adjustments were made to account for the relatively high cost of sicker patients (chapter 9).

If coverage was expanded to allow everyone to receive health insurance, then the distribution of uncompensated care would be more evenly distributed across hospitals. Hospitals would have an incentive to serve as agents in helping the uninsured obtain insurance through the state plan. As the number of uninsured Americans decreases, it may be possible to reduce or eliminate payments to public hospitals, which were more than $7 billion in 1985. As the number of uninsured decreased, the need for these subsidies would be reduced.

References

Aaron, H. 1986. "Questioning the Cost of Biomedical Research." *Health Affairs,* Summer.

Aiken, I., and Bays, K. 1984. "The Medicare Debate—Round One." *New England Journal of Medicine* 311.

Altman, S. 1987. Testimony before the Subcommittee on Health, Committee on Ways and Means, U.S. House of Representatives, February 26.

American Board of Medical Specialties. 1985. *Annual Report and Reference Handbook.* Evanston: ABMS.

American Hospital Association. A. *Annual Survey of Hospitals, 1980–86.* Chicago: AHA.

———. 1987a. *Hospital Statistics.* Chicago: AHA.

———. 1987b. *Economic Trends.* Chicago: AHA.

American Medical Association. A. *Graduate Medical Education Report, 1930–86.* Chicago: AMA.

———. B. *Survey of House Staff Stipend and Benefits, 1940–65.* Chicago: AMA.

———. C. *Directory of Residency Training Programs, 1970–88.* Chicago: AMA.

Anderson, G. 1986. "National Medical Care Spending." *Health Affairs,* Fall.

———. 1988. "Hospital Performance." Testimony before Subcommittee on Health, Committee on Ways and Means, U.S. House of Representatives, April 1.

Anderson, G., and Erickson, J. 1987. "National Medical Care Spending." *Health Affairs,* August.

Anderson, G., and Lave, J. 1985. "Financing Graduate Medical Education: Whose Responsibility?" *Health Policy,* May 28.

———. 1986. "Financing Graduate Medical Education Using Multiple Regression to Set Payment Rates." *Inquiry* 23.

Anderson, G., and Rapoza, C. 1985. "Federal Financing of Graduate Medical Education: A Proposal." *New England Journal of Medicine* 312.

Anderson, G., and Russe, C. 1987. "Biomedical Research and Technology Development." *Health Affairs,* Summer.

Anderson, G., and Steinberg, E. 1984a. "To Buy or Not to Buy: Technology Acquisition under Prospective Payment." *New England Journal of Medicine* 311.

———. 1984b. "Hospital Readmissions in the Medicare Population." *New England Journal of Medicine* 311.

————. 1986. "Prospective Payment and Nutritional Support: The Need for Reform." *Journal of Parenteral and Enteral Nutrition* 10.

Arnow, 1983. "The University's Entry Fee to Federal Research Programs." *Science* 219.

Arthur Young. 1986a. *Study of the Financing of Graduate Medical Education: Report 1.* Washington, D.C.: Arthur Young.

————. 1986b. *Study of the Financing of Graduate Medical Education: Report II.* Washington, D.C.: Arthur Young.

————. 1986c. *Study of the Financing of Graduate Medical Education: Report III.* Washington, D.C.: Arthur Young.

————. 1987. *Study of the Financing of Graduate Medical Education: Report V.* Washington, D.C.: Arthur Young.

Ashby, J. 1984. *Inequity of Medicare Prospective Payments in Large Urban Areas.* Washington, D.C.: District of Columbia Hospital Association.

Association of American Medical Colleges. 1989. *Academic Medical Centers Survey.* Washington, D.C.: AAMC.

Barocci, T. 1981. *Nonprofit Hospitals: Their Structure, Human Resources and Economic Importance.* Boston: Auburn House.

Becker, E., and Steinwald, B. 1981. "Determinants of Hospital Casemix Complexity." *Health Services Research,* Winter.

Bergen, S., and Roth, A. 1984. "Prospective Payment and the University Hospital." *New England Journal of Medicine* 310.

Berman, R., Green, J., Kwo, D., et al. 1986. "Severity of Illness and the Teaching Hospital." *Journal of Medical Education* 61.

Birnbaum, I., Hanft, R., Lave, J., et al. 1986. *Graduate Medical Education in Wisconsin.* Washington, D.C.: Lewin and Associates.

Blendon, R. 1986. "The Problems of Cost, Access and Distribution of Medical Care." *Daedalus* 115.

Bloomberg, C., Marylander, S., and Yaeger, P. 1987. "Sounding Board: Patenting Medical Technology to Promote the Progress of Science and Useful Arts." *New England Journal of Medicine* 317.

Blumenthal, D., Gluck, M., and Louis, K. 1986a. "Industrial Support of University Research in Biotechnology." *Science* 231.

————. 1986b. "University-Industry Research Relationships in Biotechnology: Implications for the University." *Science* 232.

Blumstein, J. 1986. *Uncompensated Hospital Care.* Baltimore: Johns Hopkins University Press.

Bovbjerg, R., and Koller, C. 1986. "State Health Insurance Pools: Current Performance, Future Prospect." *Inquiry* 23.

Brewster, A., Karlin, B., Hyde, L., et al. 1985. "MEDISGRPS: A Clinically Based Approach to Classifying Hospital Patients at Admission." *Inquiry* 22.

Breyer, F. 1987. "The Specification of a Hospital Cost Function: A Comment on Recent Literature." *Journal of Health Economics* 6.

Burstein, P., and Cromwell, J. 1985. "Relative Incomes and Rates of Return for U.S. Physicians." *Journal of Health Economics* 4.

Busby, D., Leming, J., and Olson, M. 1972. "Unidentified Educational Costs in a University Teaching Hospital: An Initial Study." *Journal of Medical Education* 47.

California Health Facilities. 1983. *Cost Commission Discharge Data.* Sacramento: CHF.

Cameron, J. 1985. "The Indirect Costs of Graduate Medical Education." *New England Journal of Medicine* 312.

Children's Defense Fund. 1988. Washington, D.C. Unpublished estimates.

Coffey, R., and Goldfarb, M. 1986. "DRGs and Disease Staging for Reimbursing Medicare Patients." *Medical Care* 24.

Colloton, J. 1984. "Can the American Academic Medical Center Survive?" *Johns Hopkins National Forum for Medicine,* May 9.

Commonwealth Task Force on Academic Medical Centers. 1985. *Prescription for Change.* New York: Commonwealth Fund.

Coulton, C., McClish, D., Doremus, H., Powell, S., Smookler, S., and Jackson, D. 1985. "Implications of DRG Payments for Medical Intensive Care." *Medical Care* 23.

Council of Teaching Hospitals. A. *Survey of Housestaff Stipends, Benefits, and Funding,* 1970–86. Washington, D.C.: Association of American Medical Colleges.

————. 1977. *Survey of House Staff Policy and Related Information.* Washington, D.C.: Association of American Medical Colleges.

Cowing, T., Holtman, A., and Powers, S. 1983. "Hospital Costs Analysis: A Survey and Evaluation of Recent Studies." In R. Scheffler and L. Rossiter, eds., *Advances in Health Economics and Health Services Research,* vol. 4. Greenwich: JAL Press.

Cromwell, J. 1985. "Sources of DRG Cost Variation across Urban and Rural Teaching, Non-Teaching and Large and Small Hospitals." Lexington, Mass.: Health Policy Research Consortium, Cooperative Research Center.

Davis, C. 1985. "The Impact of Prospective Payment on Clinical Research." *Journal of the American Medical Association* 253.

Davis, K., Anderson, G., Renn, S., et al. 1985. "Is Cost Containment Working?" *Health Affairs* 4.

Davis, K., and Reynolds, R. 1975. "Medicare and the Utilization of Health Care Services by the Elderly." *Journal of Human Resources* 10.

Davis, K., and Rowland, D. 1983. "Uninsured and Underserved: Inequities in Health Care in the United States." *Milbank Memorial Fund Quarterly* 61.

de Lissovoy, G., Rice, T., Gabel, J., and Gelzer, H. 1987. "Preferred Provider Organizations: One Year Later." *Inquiry* 24.

Dobson, A., and Hoy, E. 1988. "Hospital PPS Profits: Past and Prospective." *Health Affairs* 7.

Donabedian, A. 1980. *Explorations in Quality Assessment and Monitoring.* Vol. 1, *The Definition of Quality and Approaches to its Assessment.* Ann Arbor: Health Administration Press.

Eisenberg, B. 1984. "Diagnosis-Related Groups, Severity of Illness and Equitable Reimbursement under Medicare." *Journal of the American Medical Association* 251.

Employee Benefit Research Institute. 1987. *A Profile of the Non-Elderly Population Without Health Insurance.* Brief 66. Washington, D.C.: EBRI.

Enthoven, A. 1980. *Health Plan: The Only Practical Solution to the Soaring Cost of Medical Care.* Reading: Addison-Wesley.

———. 1985. Testimony before the U.S. Senate Committee on Finance. Vol. 17, *Tax Reform Proposals.* Washington, D.C.: Government Printing Office.

Etheredge, L. 1986. "Ethics and the New Insurance Market." *Inquiry* 23.

Feder, J., Hadley, J., and Zuckerman, S. 1987. "How Did Medicare's Prospective Payment System Affect Hospitals?" *New England Journal of Medicine* 317.

Feldman, R. 1976. "Some More Problems with Income-Contingent Loans: The Case of Medical Education." *Journal of Political Economy* 84.

Feldstein, M. 1971. "Hospital Cost Inflation: A Study of Nonprofit Price Dynamics." *American Economics Review* 61.

———. 1977. "Quality Change and the Demand for Hospital Care." *Econometrica* 45.

Feldstein, P., Wiekizer, T., and Wheeler, J. 1988. "Private Cost Containment." *New England Journal of Medicine* 318.

Fetter, R. 1982. *The New ICD-0-CM Diagnosis-Related Group Classification Scheme: Final Report.* New Haven: Health Systems Management Group, School of Organization and Management, Yale University.

Fitzgerald, J., et al. 1987. "Changing Patterns of Hip Fracture Care Before and After Implementation of the Prospective Payment System." *Journal of the American Medical Association* 258.

Foote, S. 1987. "Assessing Medical Technology Assessment: Past, Present, and Future." *Milbank Memorial Quarterly* 65.

Fosdick, R. 1962. *Adventure in Giving: The Story of the General Education Board, a Foundation Established by John D. Rockefeller.* New York: Harper and Row.

Frederickson, D. 1981. "Biomedical Research in the 1980s." *New England Journal of Medicine* 304.

Freeman, H., et al. 1987. "Americans Report on Their Access to Health Care." *Health Affairs,* Spring.

Friedman, B., and Shortell, S. 1988. "Financial Performance of Selected Investor-Owned and Not-for-Profit System Hospitals before and after Medicare Prospective Payment." *Health Services Research* 23.

Fruen, M., and Korper, S. 1981. "Issues In Graduate Medical Education Financing." *Journal of Health Politics, Policy and Law* 6.

Fuchs, U. 1974. *Who Shall Live? Health, Economics, and Social Choice.* New York: Basic Books.

Gabel, J., and Erman, D. 1984. "Preferred Provider Organizations: Performance, Problems, and Promise." *Health Affairs*, Spring.

Gabel, J., Jajich-Toth, C., Williams, K., Loughman, S., and Haugh, K. 1987. "The Health Industry in Transition." *Health Affairs* 6.

Garber, A., Fuchs, V., and Silverman, J. 1984. "Case Mix, Costs, and Outcomes: Differences between Faculty and Community Services in a University Hospital." *New England Journal of Medicine* 310.

Garg, M., Elkhatib, M., and Kleinberg, W. 1983. "Reimbursing for Residency Training: How Many Times?" *Medical Care* 21.

Garg, M., Elkhatib, M., Kleinberg, W., and Mulligan, J. 1982. "Reimbursing for Residency Training: How Many Times?" *Medical Care* 20.

Georgetown University Center for Health Policy, Washington, D.C. Unpublished data.

Gertman, P., and Restuccia, J. 1981. "The Appropriateness Evaluation Protocol: A Technique for Assessing Unnecessary Days of Hospital Care." *Medical Care* 19.

Ginsberg, P., and Sloan, F. 1984. "Hospital Cost Shifting." *New England Journal of Medicine* 310.

Ginzberg, E. 1982. "The Future Supply of Physicians: From Pluralism to Policy." *Health Affairs*, Fall.

Gonnella, J., Hornbrook, M., and Lewis, D. 1984. "Staging of Disease: A Case-Mix Measurement." *Journal of the American Medical Association* 251.

Gonyea, M. 1980. "Finding the Cost of Clinical Education." *Issues in Health Care*.

Gordon, N. 1988. "Minimum Health Benefits for All Workers Act." Testimony before the Subcommittee on Health and the Environment, U.S. Congress Committee on Energy and Commerce, April 15.

Grannemann, T., Brown, R., and Pauly, M. 1986. "Estimating Hospital Costs: A Multiple Output Analysis." *Journal of Health Economics* 5.

Gutterman, S., and Dobson, A. 1986. "Impact of the Medicare Prospective Payment System for Hospitals." *HCFA Review*, Spring.

Hadley, J. 1982. "Financing Graduate Medical Education: An Update and a Suggestion for Reform." *Health Policy and Education* 3.

Hadley, J. 1983a. "Medicaid Reimbursement of Teaching Hospitals." *Journal of Health Politics, Policy and Law* 7.

———. 1983b. "Teaching and Hospital Costs." *Journal of Health Economics* 2.

Hadley, J., and Feder, J. 1985. "Hospital Cost Shifting and Care for the Uninsured." *Health Affairs* 4.

Harden, V. 1986. *Inventing the NIH: Federal Biomedical Research Policy, 1887–1937.* Baltimore: Johns Hopkins University Press.

Health Care Financing Administration, Office of the Actuary, Division of National Cost Estimates, Washington, D.C. Unpublished data.

Health Insurance Association of America. 1987. Unpublished estimate. Personal communication with Dave Llewellyn.

Herdman, R. 1984. "University-Industrial Relationship." *Public Issues* 2.

Heyssel, R. 1984. "Constrained Resources in Medical Education and Research." *Health Affairs* 3.

Higham, J. 1975. *Strangers in the Land.* New York: Athenium.

Hoft, R., and Glaser, R. 1982. "The Problems and Benefits of Associating Academic Medical Center with Health Maintenance Organizations." *New England Journal of Medicine* 307.

Horn, S., Bulkley, G., Sharkey, P., Chambers, A., Horn, R., and Schramm, C. 1985. "Inter-Hospital Difference in Patient Severity Problems of Prospective Payment Based on Diagnosis-Related Groups (DRGs)." *New England Journal of Medicine* 313.

Horn, S., Horn, R., and Sharkey, P. 1984. "The Severity-of-Illness Index as a Severity Adjustment to Diagnosis-Related Groups." *Health Care Financing Review.* Annual Supplement.

Horn, S., Horn, R., Sharkey, P., et al. 1986. "Misclassification Problem in Diagnosis Groups: Cystic Fibrosis as an Example." *New England Journal of Medicine* 314.

Hornbrook, M. 1982. "Hospital Case-Mix: Its Definition and Measurement." Parts 1 and 2. *Medical Care Review* 39.

Hosek, J. 1979. *The Potential Cost Savings of Hospitals that Teach.* Santa Monica: RAND.

Hosek, J., and Massel, A. 1976. "Teaching and Hospital Costs: The Case of Radiology." Santa Monica: RAND.

Iglehart, J. 1985. "Reducing Residency Opportunities for Graduates of Foreign Medical Schools." *New England Journal of Medicine* 313.

———. 1986a. "Early Experience with Prospective Payment of Hospitals." *New England Journal of Medicine* 314.

———. 1986b. "Federal Support of Health Manpower Education." *New England Journal of Medicine* 314.

Interstudy. 1988. *Report on the HMO Industry.* Excelsior, Minn.: Interstudy.

Jencks, S., and Bobula, J. In press. "Does Accepting Referrals and Transfers Make Hospitals Expensive?" *Medical Care.*

Jencks, S., and Dobson, A. 1987. "Refining Case-Mix Measurement: The Research Evidence." *New England Journal of Medicine* 317.

Johnson, K., Rosenbaum, S., and Simons, V. 1985. *The Data Book: The Nation, States, and Cities, 1985.* Washington, D.C.: Childrens Defense Fund.

Jones, K. 1984. "The Influence of the Attending Physician on Indirect Graduate Medical Education Costs." *Journal of Medical Education* 59.

Joskow, P. 1980. "The Effects of Competition and Regulation on Hospital Bed Supply and the Reservation Quality of Hospitals." *Bell Journal of Economics* 11.

Kahn, C. 1984. "A Proposed New Role for the Insurance Industry in Biomedical Research Funding." *New England Journal of Medicine* 310.

Katz, M. 1984. "Poorhouse and the Origins of the Public Old Age Home." *Milbank Memorial Fund Quarterly* 62.

Keim, S., and Carney, M. 1975. "A Cost-Benefit Study of Selected Clinical Education Programs for Professional and Allied Health Personnel." Paper prepared for the Regional Medical Program of Texas, July 5.

Kindig, D. 1982. "A Future Shortage of Residency Training Positions?" *New England Journal of Medicine* 306.

Knowles, J., ed. 1977. *Doing Better and Feeling Worse: Health Care in the United States.* New York: Norton.

Kutina, K., Bruss, E., and Paich, M. 1985. "Impact on Academic Medical Center of Reduction in Reimbursement of Indirect Research Costs." *Journal of Medical Education* 60.

Laudicina, S. 1985. "A Comparative Survey of Medicaid Hospital Reimbursement Systems for Inpatient Services, State by State, 1980–1985." Paper prepared for the Intergovernmental Health Policy Project, George Washington University.

Lave, J. 1967. "Financing Hospital Care for the Indigent and Medically Indigent." Ph.D. diss. Harvard University.

———. 1985. "The Medicare Adjustment for the Indirect Costs of Medical Education: Historical Development and Current Status." *Association of American Medical Colleges,* January.

Lave, J., and Lave, L. 1974. *The Hospital Construction Act: An Evaluation of the Hill-Burton Programs, 1948–1973.* Washington, D.C.: American Enterprise Institute for Public Policy Research.

———. 1978. "Hospital Cost Function Analysis: Implications for Cost Controls." *Milbank Memorial Fund Quarterly* 56.

———. 1984. "Hospital Cost Functions." *Annual Review of Public Health* 5.

Lave, J., and Leinhardt, S. 1976. "The Cost and Length of a Hospital Stay." *Inquiry* 12.

Lee, R. 1984. "Subsidizing the Affluent: The Case of Medical Education." *Journal of Policy Analysis and Management* 3.

Lee, R., and Hadley, J. 1985. "The Demand for Residents." *Journal of Health Economics* 4.

Lees, D., and Rice, R. 1965. "Uncertainty and the Welfare Economics of Medical Care: Comment." *American Economic Review* 55.

Lewin, L., and Lewin, M. 1987. "Financing Charity Care in an Era of Competition." *Health Affairs* 6.

Lewis, I., and Sheps, C. 1983. *The Sick Citadel: The American Medical Center and the Public Interest.* Cambridge: Oelgeschlager, Gunn and Hain.

Lierman, T. 1983. "Health Research Funding: Politics, Promise, and Priorities." *Public Issues.*

Link, C., Long, S., and Settle, R. 1982. "Access to Medical Care under Medicaid: Differentials by Race." *Health Politics, Policy and Law* 7.

Lohr, K., Brook, R., Kamberg, C., et al. 1986. "Use of Medical Care in the Rand Health Insurance Experiment: Diagnosis- and Service-Specific Analyses in a Randomized Controlled Trial." *Medical Care* 24.

Ludmerer, K. 1985. *Learning to Heal: The Development of American Medical Education.* New York: Basic Books.

MacLeod, G., and Prussin, M. 1973. "The Continuing Evolution of Health Maintenance Organizations." *New England Journal of Medicine* 288.

MacLeod, G., Rockette, H., and Schwarz, M. 1987. "An Attitudinal Assessment of Faculty Practice Plans." *Journal of the American Medical Association* 257.

Martz, E., and Ptakowski, R. 1978. "Educational Cost to Hospitalized Patients." *Journal of Medical Education* 53.

Monheit, A., Hagan, M., and Berk, M. 1985. "The Employed Uninsured and the Role of Public Policy." *Inquiry* 22.

Mulstein, S. 1984. "The Uninsured and the Financing of Uncompensated Care: Scope, Costs, and Policy Options." *Inquiry* 21.

Munoz, E., Laughlin, A., Regan, D., Teicler, I., Margolis, I., and Wise, L. 1985. "The Financial Effects of Emergency Department Generated Admissions under Prospective Payment Systems." *Journal of the American Medical Association* 254.

Nash, D. 1987. "Graduate Medical Education: Who Will Pay How Much for What?" *Annals of Internal Medicine* 106.

National Center for Health Statistics. 1985. *Vital Statistics of the United States, 1980.* Vol. 2, *Mortality,* part A. PHS 85-1101. Washington, D.C.: Government Printing Office.

National Institutes of Health. 1984. *NIH Almanac.* Bethesda: NIH.

―――. 1989. *NIH Data Book 1988: Basic Data Relating to National Institutes of Health.* Bethesda: NIH.

Neu, C. 1976. *The Program Cost of Inpatient Care in Teaching and Nonteaching Hospitals: An Analysis of Inpatient Episodes for Medicaid Patients.* Santa Monica: RAND.

Newhouse, J. 1978. "The Structure of Health Insurance and the Erosion of Competition in the Medical Marketplace." In Greenberg, W., ed., *Competition in the Health Care Sector: Past, Present and Future.* Germantown: Aspen Systems Corporation.

―――. 1983. "Two Prospective Difficulties with Prospective Payment of Hospitals, or, It's Better to be a Resident than a Patient with a Complex Problem." *Journal of Health Economics* 2.

Newhouse, J., Manning, W., Morris, C., et al. 1981. "Some Later Results from a Controlled Trial of Cost Sharing in Health Insurance." *New England Journal of Medicine* 305.

New York State Commission on Graduate Medical Education. 1986. *Report of the New York Commission on Graduate Medical Education.* Albany: State of New York Department of Health.

Omenn, G. 1982. "Taking University Research into the Marketplace." *New England Journal of Medicine* 307.

Omen, G., and Conrad, D. 1984. "Implications of DRGs for Clinicians." *New England Journal of Medicine* 311.

Otis, G., Graham, J., and Thacker, L. 1975. "Typological Analysis of U.S. Medical Schools." *Journal of Medical Education* 50.

Payne, S. 1987. "Identifying and Managing Inappropriate Hospital Utilization." *Health Services Research* 22.

Pear, R. 1987. "Many States Are Making Health Care More Available to Uninsured People." *New York Times,* November 22.

Perry, D., Challoner, D., and Oberst, R. 1981. "Research Advances and Resource Constraints." *New England Journal of Medicine* 305.

Petersdorf, R. 1985. "A Proposal for Financing Graduate Medical Education." *New England Journal of Medicine* 312.

Peterson, C. 1986. "The Costs of Biomedical Research." *Health Affairs* 5.

Pettingill, J., and Vertrees, J. 1982. "Reliability and Validity in Hospital Case-Mix Measurement." *Health Care Financing Review* 4.

Phelps, C., and Newhouse, J. 1976. "Coinsurance, the Price of Time and the Demand for Medical Services." *Review of Economics and Statistics* 58.

Pindyck, R., and Rubinfeld, D. 1981. *Econometric Models and Economic Forecasts.* New York: McGraw-Hill.

ProPAC (Prospective Payment Assessment Commission). 1987. *Medicare Prospective Payment and the American Health Care System.* Report to Congress. Washington, D.C.: Government Printing Office.

———. 1988a. *Report and Recommendations to the Secretary, U.S. Department of Health and Human Services.* Washington, D.C.: Government Printing Office.

———. 1988b. *Technical Approaches to the Report and Recommendations to the Secretary.* Washington, D.C.: Government Printing Office.

Reed, W., Cawley, K., and Anderson, R. 1986. "The Effect of a Public Hospital's Transfer Policy on Patient Care." *New England Journal of Medicine* 315.

Relman, A. 1984. "Are Teaching Hospitals Worth the Extra Cost?" *New England Journal of Medicine* 310.

———. 1985. "Dealing with Conflicts of Interest." *New England Journal of Medicine* 313.

Reuben, D. 1984. "Learning Diagnostic Restraint." *New England Journal of Medicine* 310.

Rice, D. 1964. "Coverage of the Aged and their Hospital Utilization in 1962." *Social Security Bulletin* 27.

Robert Wood Johnson Foundation. 1982. *Affordable Health Care Programs.* Princeton: RWJ Foundation.

Robinson, J., and Luft, H. 1987. "Competition and the Cost of Hospital Care: 1972–1982." *Journal of the American Medical Association* 257.

Rogers, D. 1978. *American Medicine Challenge for the 1980s.* Cambridge: Ballinger.

Rogers, D., Blendon, R., and Maloney, T. 1982. "Who Needs Medicaid?" *New England Journal of Medicine* 307.

Rosner, D. 1982. "Health Care for the Truly Needy: Nineteenth Century Origins of the Concept." *Milbank Memorial Fund Quarterly* 30.

Russell, L. 1979. *Technology and Hospitals*. Washington, D.C.: Brookings.

Ruther, M., and Dobson, A. 1981. "Equal Treatment and Unequal Benefits; A Reexamination of the Use of Medicare Services by Race, 1967–1976." *Health Care Financing Review 2*.

Salkever, D., and Bice, R. 1976. "The Impact of Certificate-of-Need on Hospital Investment." *Milbank Memorial Fund Quarterly 54*.

Salkever, D., Steinwachs, D., and Rapp, A. 1985. "Hospital Cost and Efficiency under per Service and per Case Payment in Maryland: A Tale of the Carrot and the Stick." *Inquiry 23*.

Schiff, R., Ansell, D., Schlosser, J., et al. 1986. "Transfers to a Public Hospital." *New England Journal of Medicine 314*.

Schleiter, M., and Tarlov, A. 1985. "National Study of Internal Medicine Manpower: IX. Internal Medicine Residency and Fellowship Training: 1984 Update." *Annals of Internal Medicine 102*.

Schroeder, S., and O'Leary, D. 1977. "Differences in Laboratory Use and Length of Stay between University and Community Hospitals." *Journal of Medical Education 52*.

Schwartz, W., Newhouse, J., and Williams, A. 1985. "Is the Teaching Hospital an Endangered Species?" *New England Journal of Medicine 313*.

Sheingold, S. 1988. "Alternatives for Using Multivariate Regressions to Adjust Medicare's Prospective Payment Rates." Washington, D.C.: Congressional Budget Office.

Shryock, R., and Oki, I. 1951. *The Development of Modern Medicine*. Tokyo: Sogensha.

Sloan, F., Feldman, R., and Steinwald, A. 1983. "Effects of Teaching on Hospital Costs." *Journal of Health Economics 2*.

Sloan, F., Valvona, J., and Mullner, R. 1986. "Identifying the Issues: A Statistical Profile." In Sloan, F., Blumstein, J., and Perrin, J., eds., *Uncompensated Hospital Care: Rights and Responsibilities*. Baltimore: Johns Hopkins University Press.

Smith, C. 1986. "Health Care Delivery System Changes: A Special Challenge for Teaching Hospitals." *Journal of Medical Education 60*.

Smith, J. 1975. "Allied Health Program Costing in a Medical Center." *Journal of Applied Health 4*.

Somers, H., and Somers, A. 1967. *Medicare and the Hospitals: Issues and Prospects*. Washington, D.C.: Brookings.

Starr, P. 1982. *The Social Transformation of American Medicine*. New York: Basic Books.

State of Texas. 1987. Texas Department of Health, Article 4437f, Vernons Texas Civil Statutes sec. 5(a) 25, Texas Administrative Code sec. 133.21 ch. 11: Rules Governing Hospital Patient Transferring Policies, subsection 5b of Hospital Licensing Standards.

Steinberg, E., and Anderson, G. 1987. "Potential 'Losers' under per Case Payment." *Annals of Internal Medicine 106*.

Stern, R., and Epstein, A. 1985. "Institutional Responses to Prospective Payment Based on Diagnosis Related Groups." *New England Journal of Medicine* 312.

Stevens, R. 1974. *Welfare Medicine in America. A Case Study of Medicaid.* New York: Free Press.

———. 1978. "Graduate Medical Education: A Continuing History." *Journal of Medical Education* 53.

———. 1982. "A Poor Sort of Memory: Voluntary Hospitals and Government before the Depression." *Milbank Memorial Fund Quarterly* 60.

Stimmel, B., and Benenson, T. 1979. "United States Citizens in Foreign Medical Schools and the Future Supply of Physicians." *New England Journal of Medicine* 300.

Strickland, S. 1972. *Politics, Science and the Dread Disease.* Cambridge: Harvard University Press.

Sulvetta, M. 1985. "Dimensions of the Uncompensated Care Problem." In *Uncompensated Hospital Care: Issues and Options.* Brandeis University Health Policy Consortium, March.

Sulvetta, M., and Swartz, K. 1986. *The Uninsured and Uncompensated Care: A Chart Book.* Washington, D.C.: National Health Policy Forum.

Swartz, K. 1988. "The Uninsured and Workers without Employee Group Health Insurance." Working Paper 3789-02. Washington, D.C.: Urban Institute.

Tarlov, A., Schleiter, M., Weil, P., and the Association of Professors of Medicine Task Force on Manpower. 1979. "National Study of Internal Medicine Manpower: IV. Residency and Fellowship Training 1977–1978." *Annals of Internal Medicine* 91.

Thorpe, K. 1988a. "The Use of Regression Analysis to Determine Hospital Payment: The Case of Medicare's Indirect Teaching Adjustment." *Inquiry* 25.

———. 1988b. "Why Are Urban Hospital Costs So High? The Relative Importance of Admissions, Teaching, Competition and Case-Mix." *Health Services Research* 22.

Tierney, T. 1969. "Medicare and the Financing of Teaching Hospitals." *Journal of Medical Education* 44.

U.S. Bureau of the Census. 1986. *Current Population Survey: 1986.* Hyattsville: Bureau of the Census.

U.S. Congress, Congressional Budget Office. 1979. *Effect of PSROs on Health Care Costs: Current Findings and Future Evaluation.* Washington, D.C.: Government Printing Office.

———. 1985. *Indirect Teaching Adjustment for Medicare's Prospective Payment System: Issues and Options.* Washington, D.C.: Government Printing Office.

———. 1987. *Reducing the Deficit: Spending Reserve Options. A Report to the Senate and House Committees on the Budget, Part II.* Washington, D.C.: Government Printing Office.

U.S. Congress, Office of Technology Assessment. 1984. *Medical Technology and the Costs of the Medical Program.* Washington, D.C.: Government Printing Office.

U.S. Department of Health and Human Services. 1980. *Graduate Medical Education, National Advisory Committee Summary Report.* Vol. 1. Washington, D.C.: Government Printing Office.

———. 1981a. *The 1981 Short-Term, General, and Other Special Hospital Civil Rights Survey.* Washington, D.C.: Government Printing Office.

———. 1981b. *Medicare 1981 Cost Report File.* Baltimore: Health Care Financing Administration.

———. 1981c. *The 1980 National Medical Care Utilization and Expenditure Survey of the Civilian and Non-Institutionalized.* Rockville: National Center for Health Services Research.

———. 1984. *NIH Almanac.* Bethesda: National Institutes of Health.

———. 1985. *NIH Research Awards Index.* Bethesda: National Institutes of Health.

———. 1986a. *The 1986 Short-Term, General, and Other Special Hospital Civil Rights Survey.* Washington, D.C.: Government Printing Office.

———. 1986b. *Compendium of State Health. Distribution Programs.* ODAM Report 2-87. Washington, D.C.: Government Printing Office.

———. 1987. *NIH Data Book 1987: Basic Data Relating to National Institutes of Health.* Bethesda: National Institutes of Health.

U.S. General Accounting Office. 1985. *Information Requirements for Evaluating the Impacts of Medicare's Prospective Payment on Post Hospital Long-term Care Services: Preliminary Report.* GAO/PEMD-85-8. Washington, D.C.: Government Printing Office.

U.S. Senate. 1983. *Social Security Amendments of 1983.* Report 98—23. Washington, D.C.: Government Printing Office.

———. 1985. *Americans at Risk: The Case of the Medically Uninsured.* Report 99-6. Washington, D.C.: Government Printing Office.

Waldo, D., Lewit, K., and Lazenby, H. 1986. "National Health Expenditures, 1985." *Health Care Financing Review* 8.

Wilensky, G. 1984. "Solving Uncompensated Hospital Care: Targeting the Indigent and the Uninsured." *Health Affairs* 3.

———. 1986. "Underwriting the Uninsured: Targeting Providers or Individuals?" In Sloan, F., Blumstein, J., and Perrin, J., eds., *Uncompensated Hospital Care: Rights and Responsibilities.* Baltimore: Johns Hopkins University Press.

Wilensky, G., and Berk, M. 1982. "The Health Care of the Poor and the Role of Medicaid." *Health Affairs* 1.

Wrenn, K. 1985. "No Insurance, No Admission." *New England Journal of Medicine* 312.

Yoder, S. 1977. *Methods for Determining the Cost of Graduate Medical Ed-*

ucation. Washington, D.C.: Research Associate Institute of Medicine, Division of Health Manpower and Resources Development.

Young, W., et al. 1983. *Hospital Case-Mix Development and Implementation.* Pittsburgh: Health Care Research Department, Blue Cross of Western Pennsylvania.

Index

Page numbers in italics indicate material in figures or tables.

About the Authors

Gerard F. Anderson is director of the Center for Hospital Finance and Management, codirector of the Program for Medical Technology and Practice Assessment, and associate professor of health policy and management at the Johns Hopkins University.

Judith R. Lave is professor of health economics at the University of Pittsburgh.

Catherine M. Russe is an associate at Booz, Allen & Hamilton.

Patricia Neuman is a professional staff member on the Ways and Means Committee, U.S. House of Representatives.

Providing Hospital Services

Typeset in ITC Caslon 224 by
Brevis Press, Bethany, Conn.,
from a design by
S. Stoneham, Studio 1812, Baltimore, Md.
Printed on 50-lb. Glatfelter B-16 by
Thomson-Shore, Inc., Dexter, Mich.